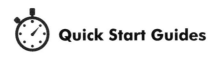

CW00410169

The Essential
800 CALORIE
MEDITERRANEAN DIET
15 Minute Meals

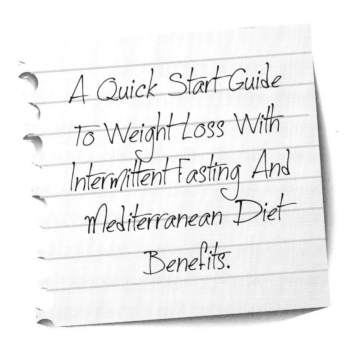

A Quick Start Guide To Weight Loss With Intermittent Fasting And Mediterranean Diet Benefits.

Delicious Calorie-Counted 15 Minute Meals

First published in 2020 by Erin Rose Publishing

Text and illustration copyright © 2020 Erin Rose Publishing

Design: Julie Anson

ISBN: 978-1-9161523-5-9

A CIP record for this book is available from the British Library.

DISCLAIMER: This book is for informational purposes only and not intended as a substitute for the medical advice, diagnosis or treatment of a physician or qualified healthcare provider. The reader should consult a physician before undertaking a new health care regime and in all matters relating to his/her health, and particularly with respect to any symptoms that may require diagnosis or medical attention.

While every care has been taken in compiling the recipes for this Book we cannot accept responsibility for any problems which arise as a result of preparing one of the recipes. The author and publisher disclaim responsibility for any adverse effects that may arise from the use or application of the recipes in this book. Some of the recipes in this book include nuts. If you have a nut allergy it's important to avoid these.

CONTENTS

Recipes

Breakfast Recipes

Lunch Recipes

Dinner Recipes

Desserts, Treats & Snacks Recipes

INTRODUCTION

If you are intermittent fasting (IF) and need some fast, easy, calorie-counted, Mediterranean style recipes, to achieve great weight loss results that fit into your busy lifestyle, then look no further!

Even if you're short on time you can still make delicious, mouth-watering foods suitable for the 800 calorie diet, a low calorie or Mediterranean diet which gives you optimum weight loss and health.

Bringing together the world's most successful diets, this easy-to-use cookbook provides you with delicious recipes for fast, healthy weight loss. Low calorie, low carb is beneficial for anyone who wants to lose weight and improve their health.

In this **Quick Start Guide** we bring you calorie counted recipes which are easy and concise, so you can enjoy them even with a busy lifestyle. There are so many fast and tasty recipes to choose from you can add variety into your diet without spending too much time in the kitchen. If you are ready to improve your health, read on!

The Mediterranean Diet has been shown to provide health benefits, reducing cholesterol, improving longevity, reducing blood pressure, the risk of heart disease, strokes, diabetes, blood sugar levels, inflammation and obesity.

Amazing weight loss success has been achieved through Intermittent fasting on the 5:2 diet with thousands getting to their goal weight by significantly restricting their calorie intake 2 days a week. Now, research shows the optimum number of calories you can consume and still lose weight is 800 calories per day. Even better! Team that with the health benefits of Mediterranean style food and you have a winner!

For all the essential information and quick, calorie-counted recipes which help prevent hunger while losing weight, read on!

Achieving Optimum Weight Loss On 800 Calories

A study by Oxford University in which an overweight group replaced meals with soups, shakes and bars which totalled 800 calories per day, showed health markers and an improvement in cardiovascular and metabolic health plus an average 10kg weight loss

Overweight type 2 diabetics who followed an 800-calorie-a-day diet for 12 weeks 'reversed' their diabetes, achieved and sustained average weight loss of 10kg according to a study by Newcastle University.

A daily limit of 800 calories is a lot less than the recommended intake to maintain weight, which for a woman, which is 2000 calories and for a man is 2,500 calories.

Simply put, the 800 calorie diet plan involves restricting calories, on a daily basis, for no more than 12 weeks. Or following the 5:2 diet plan by consuming up to 800 calories 2 days a week, whilst eating a normal healthy diet for the 5 days.

Such calorie restriction is safe and achievable for most people. Against popular belief, fast weight loss can be maintained, lower blood sugar levels, in some cases even reversing pre-diabetes and type 2 diabetes.

By restricting calories you will be reducing, or cutting out, junk food, including refined carbohydrates, sugars and harmful fats on fasting days whilst eating vegetables, healthy fats and quality protein. This will have beneficial changes on the health of your gut too.

Eating low carbohydrate foods improves blood sugar, reduces your waistline and boosts your health. Blood sugar rises every time we eat, even more so from rapidly absorbed sugars and starchy carbohydrates. It later falls, when the quick effect of the quickly absorbed food wears off, causing peaks and troughs in the blood sugar causing hunger, fatigue and cravings for more sugar. To prevent huge swings in your blood sugar it is best to avoid starchy carbohydrates, sugar and alcohol in order to stabilise the body.

Another popular and proven successful weight loss technique is Time Restricted Eating (TRE). This means eating all calories within a certain time frame each day. Often this can be a window of 8 to 16 hours a day, stretching the overnight fasting period, so you would consume no calories during this time. Time restricted allows the body to repair and you can start with a shorter fasting time and gradually increase it.

The benefits of calorie restriction and intermittent fasting extends beyond weight loss, and it is suitable for most people who are overweight. However, check with your doctor or health care professional that it is safe for you to do so before you begin.

Fasting is not suitable for the elderly, convalescing, children, during pregnancy or breastfeeding, or if you suffer from or have a history of an eating disorder or have a low BMI or have other medical conditions. Always seek your doctor's advice and especially regarding medication changes.

How To Get Started

Beginning any diet can be daunting so allow yourself to do it in whatever way works best for you, depending on how much weight you have to lose and how quickly you wish to shed extra pounds. Decide which weight loss approach to take.

You can:
1. **Restrict yourself to 800 calories a day for 2 weeks and up to a maximum of 12 weeks.**

2. **Follow the 5:2 diet, restricting yourself to 800 calories for 2 days a week and eating sensibly for 5 days.**

3. **Combine fasting and/or non-fasting days with time restricted eating. This means all food should be eaten in an 8–12 hour window each day.**

Plan which days you are fasting so you can be prepared. Increase your fluid intake on these days. Not only will it replace your usual food intake it will help your body eliminate fat. Drinking 2-3 litres a day is advisable.

Avoiding processed foods, sugar and carbohydrates such as pasta, bread, biscuits, cakes, cereals, crackers, noodles, rice and potatoes. Beware of sugary sauces like sweet chilli, BBQ, ketchup and concentrated fruit juices or fast food containing hidden sugars. Processed food are often contain high amounts of sugar and fat and it's thought that combination is what causes cravings for junk food and results in weight gain.

Familiarise yourself with what you can eat and remove tempting foods from your cupboards.

You can eat your daily calorie limit over 2 or 3 meals, depending on what suits you and fits in with your lifestyle. Some prefer to extend their overnight fasting by having a late breakfast and early evening meal as they find it easier. However, you can spread your calorie intake over breakfast, lunch and dinner, opting for lighter meals.

This may take a little experimenting and adapting as you begin your diet and work out what works best for you.

You choose to stick to 800 calories a day for 14 days, or however long you decide, depending on how rapidly you want to lose weight and then switch to the 5:2 diet. Eating low carbohydrate foods will reduce any cravings or hunger pangs making it much easier for you. Eating protein will help you feel satiated for longer.

The recipes are all calorie counted and listed according to their calorie content. This will make it easy to select what to have for each meal. You can choose whether to have 2 or 3 meals a day. The recipes can be used for whichever meal you choose – just stay within the 800 calorie total on fasting days.

This cookbook also contains recipes for healthy, low-carb, low-calorie desserts, however only eat these in moderation and avoid them completely if you have sugar cravings. These can be reduced or eliminated completely by avoiding sugar and starchy carbohydrates.

Diet Tips

- **Keep a food diary. Writing down what you eat helps you track your calorie consumption and you can also log how you are feeling, including energy, sleep, weight loss and fluid intake. It's great to reflect and see how you're doing.**

- **Decide when the best time to fast is. Avoiding social get-togethers, holidays and weekends will help you kick start your plan.**

- **On non-fasting days, don't binge. You can stick to the low carb recipes and don't over-do the portions.**

- **Staying busy will help take your mind off food, especially when you first start. Get up and do something. Exercise helps, even if it's going for a walk.**

- **You can fill up on high volume foods like broccoli, cauliflower, carrots and heaps of lettuce or spinach without adding large amounts of calories.**

- **At mealtimes, replace starchy carbohydrates with lots of veggies and you'll feel less sluggish and hungry.**

- Schedule in easy meals, plan in advance so you avoid temptation. That way you can also avoid missing a meal.

- Drink plenty of water!

- Prepare some tasty meals and snacks for the fridge or freezer and plan ahead so you aren't tempted to overdo the calories.

- Finding a diet buddy is not only god for moral but you can also swap ideas, recipes and provide encouragement.

You must always seek the advice of your doctor for any health issues and especially to make sure there are no underlying conditions. This diet is beneficial to most people however always check with your medical advisor or doctor before embarking on any dietary changes, especially if you are diabetic or are on medication which may need to be monitored or adjusted

Top Tips For Fast Easy Cooking

Make good use of leftover food and you can create a quick and tasty omelette, stir-fry or soup without any fuss. Eggs add so much variety with omelettes and scrambles and they add protein if you don't have meat available.

Chopping vegetables and meats into smaller pieces will reduce the cooking time. Improvise with your ingredients. If you don't have a particular ingredient in the cupboard, make a substitution for something similar, like kale instead of spinach.

Keep an abundant supply of key ingredients as store cupboard essentials, such as tinned and frozen goods. Ready cooked pulses and beans, tinned tomatoes, tuna, stock (broth) and vegetables are a great resource and backup if your fridge is getting low. Yes, fresh is best but frozen vegetables are a great substitute without losing too many of nutrients.

Batch looking larger portions of a meal which can be stored in the freezer means you can save time later with a quick healthy meal which can be defrosted. Remember to label your freezer bags or containers so you can easily identify the contents.

Pre-prepared vegetables which have been washed, peeled and chopped ready for cooking are handy to have in the fridge although some find the taste is not quite the same.

Ready cooked chicken and meat bought from the supermarket means you can literally assemble a meal using salad leaves or add it to soups and stir-fries to save time.

Mason jars are not only a great way of storing and transporting foods such as carrying salads to work, they can also be put in the microwave to warm up lunches.

BREAKFAST RECIPES

Avocado & Banana Smoothie

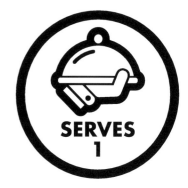

SERVES 1

233
calories
per serving

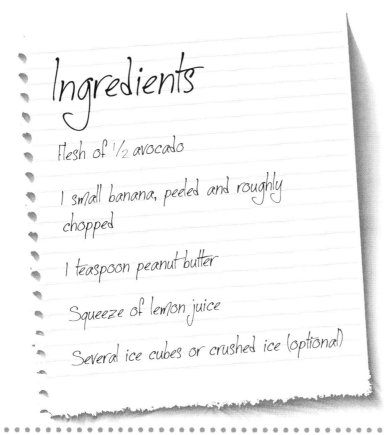

Ingredients

Flesh of ½ avocado

1 small banana, peeled and roughly chopped

1 teaspoon peanut butter

Squeeze of lemon juice

Several ice cubes or crushed ice (optional)

Method

Place all of the ingredients into a blender and blitz until smooth. If your blender doesn't tolerate ice you can just add a few cubes.

Coffee & Nut Butter Protein Shake

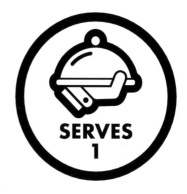

Ingredients

250mls (8fl oz) milk (or milk alternative)

1 teaspoon instant coffee powder

1 teaspoon smooth peanut butter

¼ teaspoon stevia sweetener (optional)

1 tablespoon vanilla whey protein powder (sugar-free)

Several ice cubes

SERVES 1

224 calories per serving

Method

Place all of the ingredients into blender or food processor and blitz until smooth. Serve into a glass and enjoy!

11

Chocolate Protein Shake

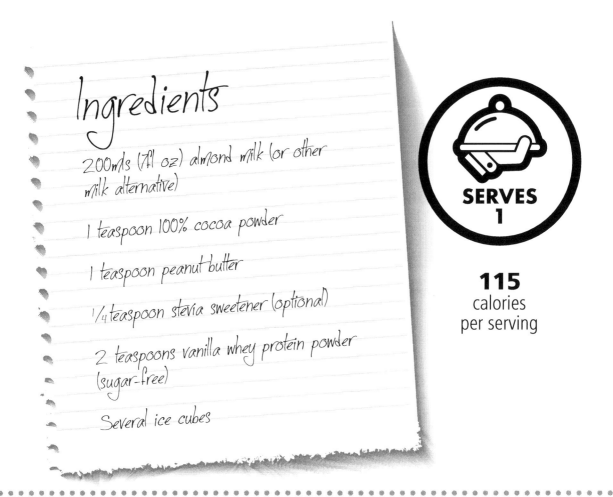

Ingredients

200mls (7fl oz) almond milk (or other milk alternative)

1 teaspoon 100% cocoa powder

1 teaspoon peanut butter

1/4 teaspoon stevia sweetener (optional)

2 teaspoons vanilla whey protein powder (sugar-free)

Several ice cubes

SERVES 1

115 calories per serving

Method

Place all of the ingredients into blender or food processor and blitz until smooth. Serve into a glass and enjoy!

Summer Berry Smoothie

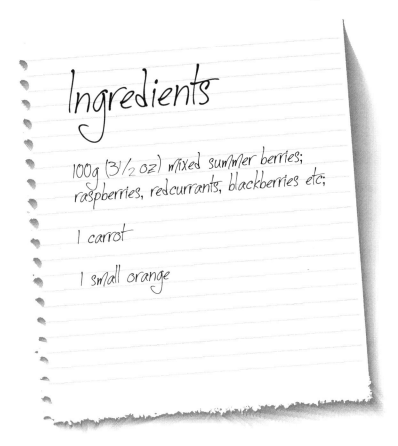

Ingredients

100g (3½ oz) mixed summer berries; raspberries, redcurrants, blackberries etc;

1 carrot

1 small orange

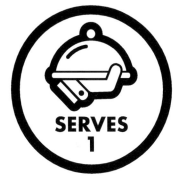

SERVES 1

107 calories per serving

Method

Place all the ingredients into a blender with enough water to cover them and process until smooth.

Strawberry & Avocado Smoothie

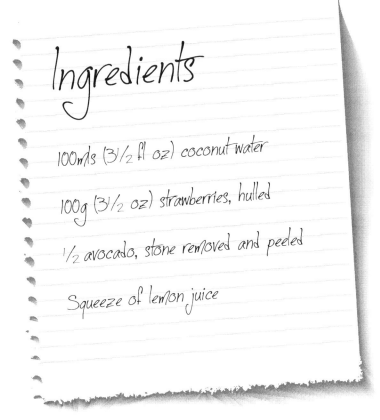

Ingredients

100mls (3½ fl oz) coconut water

100g (3½ oz) strawberries, hulled

½ avocado, stone removed and peeled

Squeeze of lemon juice

**SERVES
1**

187
calories
per serving

Method

Toss all of the ingredients into a food processor and blitz until smooth and creamy. You can add a little water if you like it less thick.

Apple & Ginger Smoothie

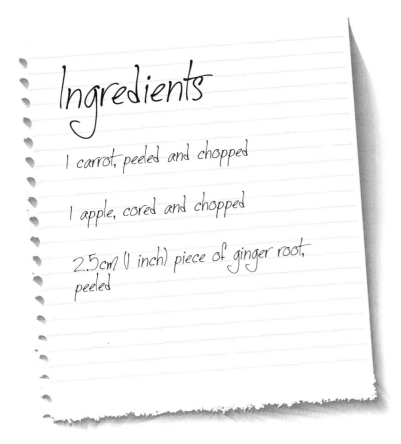

Ingredients

1 carrot, peeled and chopped

1 apple, cored and chopped

2.5cm (1 inch) piece of ginger root, peeled

**SERVES
1**

84
calories
per serving

Method

Place all of the ingredients into a blender with enough water to cover them. Blitz until smooth. Serve and drink straight away.

Detox Smoothie

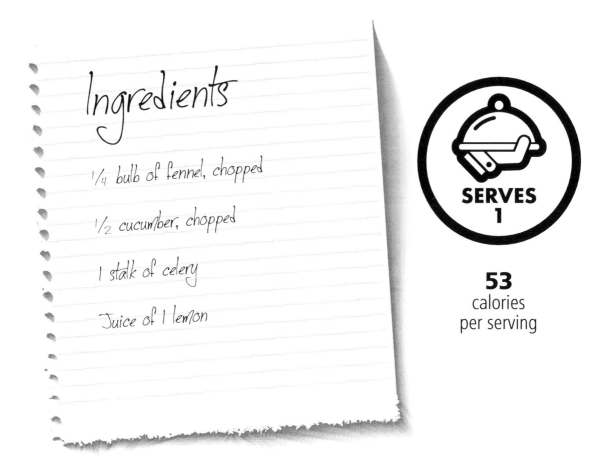

Ingredients

¼ bulb of fennel, chopped

½ cucumber, chopped

1 stalk of celery

Juice of 1 lemon

SERVES 1

53 calories per serving

Method

Place the fennel, cucumber and celery into a food processor or smoothie maker and add the lemon juice together with enough water to cover the ingredients. Process until smooth.

Apple & Lime Shots

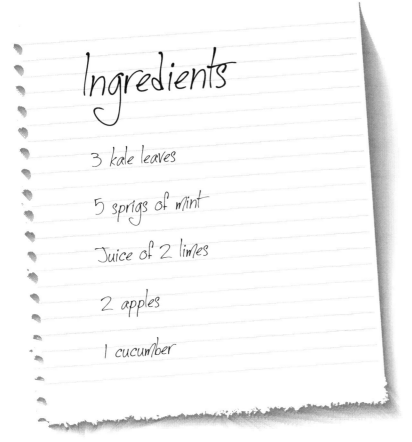

Ingredients

3 kale leaves

5 sprigs of mint

Juice of 2 limes

2 apples

1 cucumber

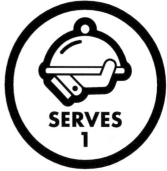

**SERVES
1**

152
calories
per serving

Method

Place the lime juice, apples, cucumber, kale and mint into a juicer and extract the juice. Alternatively, use a blender and add sufficient water to cover the ingredients. Store in a bottle in the fridge. You can take healthy shots throughout the day or you can just drink it all straight away.

Kiwi Salad Shots

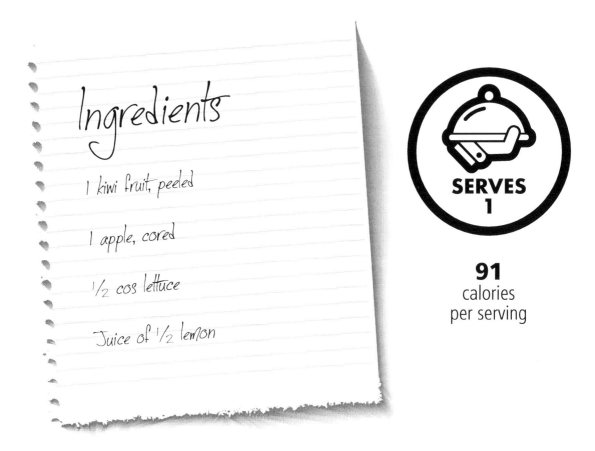

Ingredients

1 kiwi fruit, peeled

1 apple, cored

½ cos lettuce

Juice of ½ lemon

**SERVES
1**

91
calories
per serving

Method

Place all of the ingredients into a food processor with just enough water to cover them. Blitz until smooth. Pour the liquid into a glass bottle and keep it in the fridge, ready for you to have fresh shots throughout the day and a healthy drink between meals. Alternatively you can just drink it all straight away.

Pear Salad Smoothie

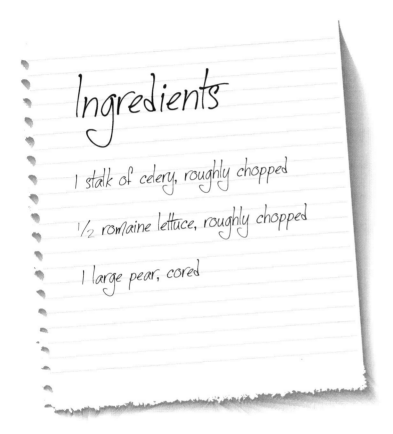

Ingredients

1 stalk of celery, roughly chopped

1/2 romaine lettuce, roughly chopped

1 large pear, cored

**SERVES
1**

83
calories
per serving

Method

Place all of the ingredients into a blender with sufficient water to cover them and blitz until smooth.

Raspberry & Cashew Nut Crunch

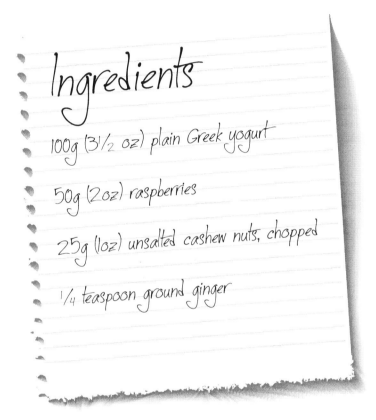

Ingredients

100g (3½ oz) plain Greek yogurt

50g (2oz) raspberries

25g (1oz) unsalted cashew nuts, chopped

¼ teaspoon ground ginger

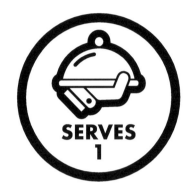

SERVES
1

291
calories
per serving

Method

Mash together half of the raspberries and all of the ginger with the yogurt. Using a glass, place a layer of yogurt with half of the remaining raspberries and a sprinkling of chopped cashews, followed by another layer of the same until you reach the top of the glass.

Savoury Mug Muffin

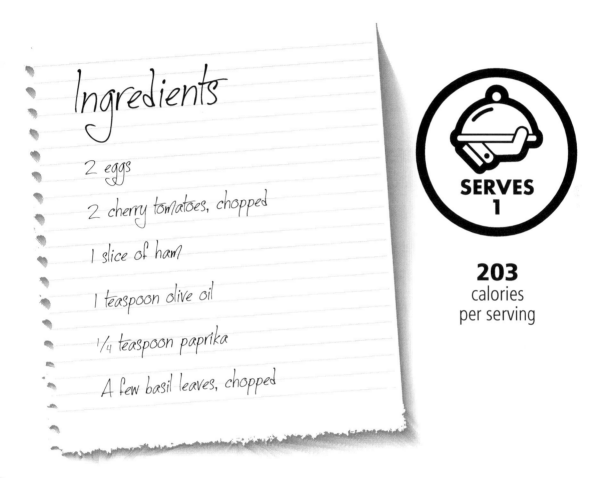

Ingredients

2 eggs

2 cherry tomatoes, chopped

1 slice of ham

1 teaspoon olive oil

¼ teaspoon paprika

A few basil leaves, chopped

SERVES 1

203 calories per serving

Method

Crack the eggs into a large mug and beat them. Add in the olive oil, ham, tomato, basil and paprika and mix well. Place the mug in a microwave and cook on full power for 30 seconds. Stir and return it to the microwave for another 30 seconds, stir and cook for another 30-60 seconds or until the egg is set. Serve it in the mug. Experiment with other ingredients, like chicken, prawns, bacon, beef, cheese, spring onions (scallions) and herbs.

Herby Mushroom Omelette

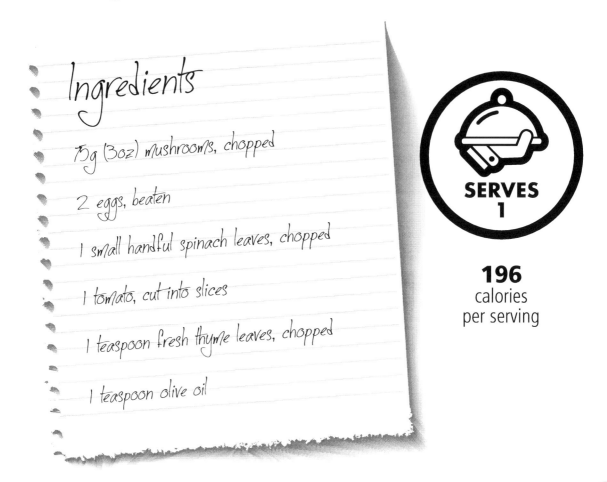

Ingredients

75g (3oz) mushrooms, chopped

2 eggs, beaten

1 small handful spinach leaves, chopped

1 tomato, cut into slices

1 teaspoon fresh thyme leaves, chopped

1 teaspoon olive oil

SERVES 1

196 calories per serving

Method

Heat the olive oil in a saucepan, add the mushrooms and cook until softened. Remove them and set aside. Pour the beaten eggs into the frying pan and allow them to set. Transfer the omelette to a plate and fill it with the mushrooms, spinach, tomato and herbs then fold it over. Enjoy.

Raspberry & Lemon Swirl

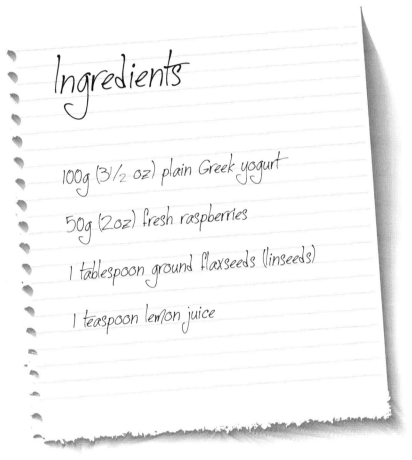

Ingredients

100g (3½ oz) plain Greek yogurt

50g (2oz) fresh raspberries

1 tablespoon ground flaxseeds (linseeds)

1 teaspoon lemon juice

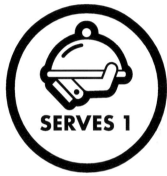

SERVES 1

208
calories
per serving

Method

Place the raspberries into blender or food processor and blitz to a smooth purée. Place the yogurt into a bowl and mix in the flaxseeds (linseeds) and lemon juice. Add the raspberry purée and partly stir it in leaving swirls in the yogurt. Serve and enjoy.

Poached Eggs & Spinach

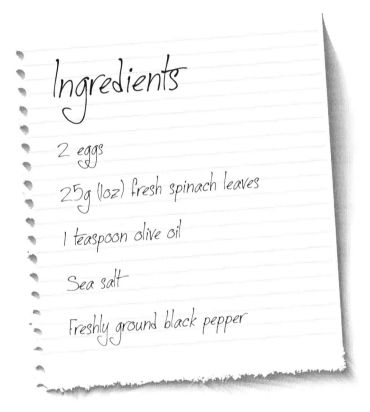

Ingredients

2 eggs

25g (1oz) fresh spinach leaves

1 teaspoon olive oil

Sea salt

Freshly ground black pepper

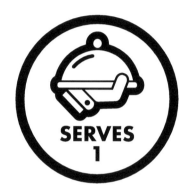

**SERVES
1**

178
calories
per serving

Method

Scatter the spinach leaves onto a plate and drizzle the olive oil over them. Bring a shallow pan of water to the boil, add in the eggs and cook until the whites become firm. Serve the eggs on top of the spinach and season with salt and pepper.

Herby Mediterranean Scramble

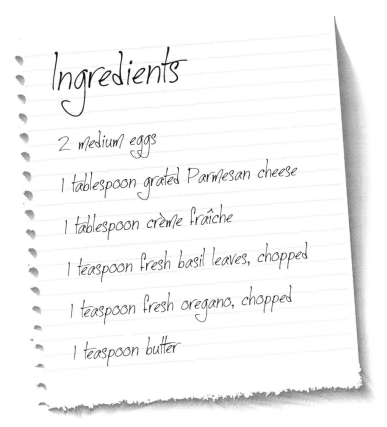

Ingredients

2 medium eggs

1 tablespoon grated Parmesan cheese

1 tablespoon crème fraîche

1 teaspoon fresh basil leaves, chopped

1 teaspoon fresh oregano, chopped

1 teaspoon butter

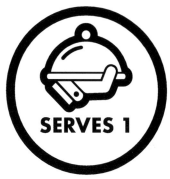

SERVES 1

204
calories
per serving

Method

Crack the eggs into a bowl, whisk them up. Add in the Parmesan cheese, crème fraîche, basil and oregano. Heat the butter in a frying pan. Pour in the egg mixture and stir constantly until the eggs are scrambled and set. Serve and enjoy.

Coconut & Lemon Yogurt

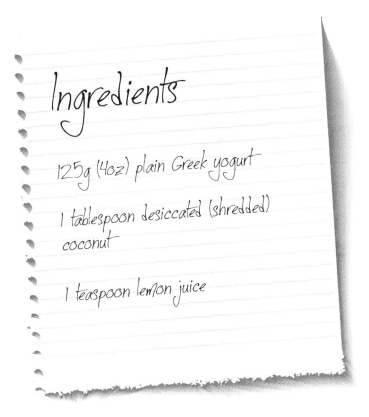

Ingredients

125g (4oz) plain Greek yogurt

1 tablespoon desiccated (shredded) coconut

1 teaspoon lemon juice

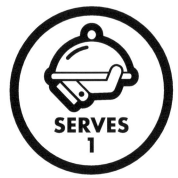

**SERVES
1**

258
calories
per serving

Method

Place the yogurt in a serving bowl and stir in the coconut and lemon juice and stir well. Serve into a bowl and eat straight away.

Chocolate
& Macadamia Yogurt

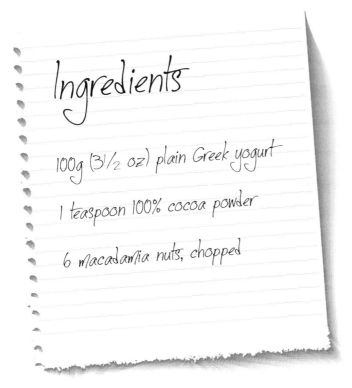

Ingredients

100g (3½ oz) plain Greek yogurt

1 teaspoon 100% cocoa powder

6 macadamia nuts, chopped

SERVES 1

227
calories
per serving

Method

Place the yogurt and cocoa powder into a bowl and stir until completely combined. Sprinkle the chopped nuts over the top. Serve and enjoy!

LUNCH RECIPES

Prawn & Basil Savoury Muffin

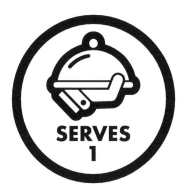

SERVES 1

216 calories per serving

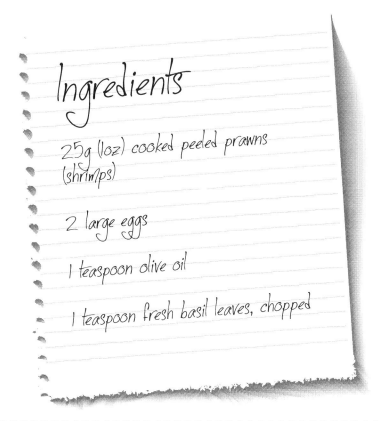

Ingredients

25g (1oz) cooked peeled prawns (shrimps)

2 large eggs

1 teaspoon olive oil

1 teaspoon fresh basil leaves, chopped

Method

Crack the eggs into a large mug and beat them. Add in the oil, prawns (shrimps) and basil. Place the mug in a microwave and cook on full power for 30 seconds. Stir and return it to the microwave for another 30 seconds, stir and cook for another 30-60 seconds or until the egg is set. Serve it in the mug.

Cheese & Olive Frittata

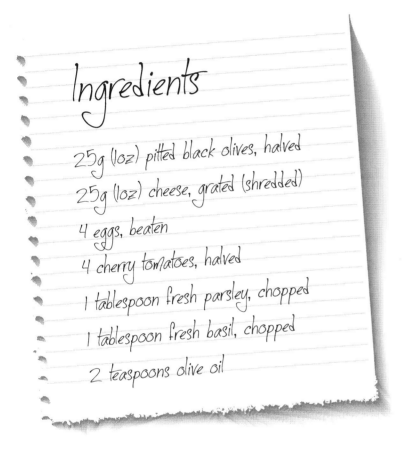

Ingredients

25g (1oz) pitted black olives, halved

25g (1oz) cheese, grated (shredded)

4 eggs, beaten

4 cherry tomatoes, halved

1 tablespoon fresh parsley, chopped

1 tablespoon fresh basil, chopped

2 teaspoons olive oil

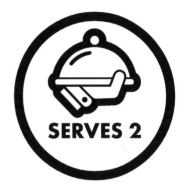

SERVES 2

249
calories
per serving

Method

Whisk the eggs in a bowl and add in the parsley, basil, olives and tomatoes. Stir in the cheese. Heat the oil in a small frying pan and pour in the egg mixture. Cook until the egg mixture completely sets. You can finish it off under a hot grill (broiler) if you wish. Gently remove it from the pan and cut it into two. You can easily double the quantity of ingredients and store the extra portions to be eaten cold.

Chorizo Scramble

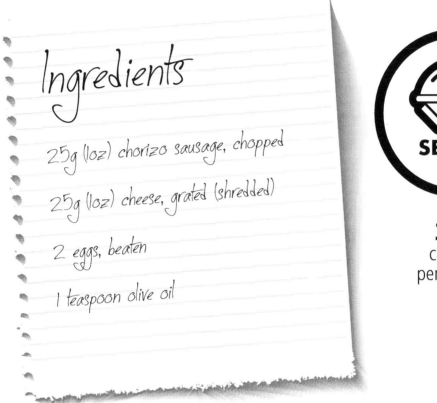

Ingredients

25g (1oz) chorizo sausage, chopped

25g (1oz) cheese, grated (shredded)

2 eggs, beaten

1 teaspoon olive oil

SERVES 1

379 calories per serving

Method

Heat the oil in a frying pan and add in the chorizo. Cook for around 2 minutes. Pour in the beaten egg and stir, scrambling the eggs until completely cooked. Serve onto a plate and sprinkle with grated (shredded) cheese.

Parmesan Asparagus

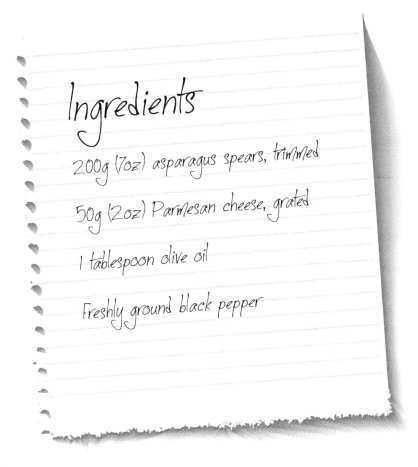

Ingredients

200g (7oz) asparagus spears, trimmed

50g (2oz) Parmesan cheese, grated

1 tablespoon olive oil

Freshly ground black pepper

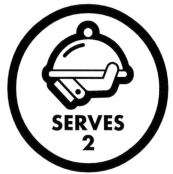

SERVES 2

191
calories
per serving

Method

Heat the olive oil in a frying pan or griddle pan, add the asparagus and cook for around 4 minutes, turning occasionally. Sprinkle the parmesan cheese on top of the asparagus and cook for another couple of minutes or until the cheese has softened. Serve and season with black pepper. Eat straight away, either on its own, or with a leafy green salad.

Quick Red Pepper & Basil Soup

Ingredients

4 red peppers (Bell peppers), deseeded and chopped

3 cloves of garlic, crushed

1 onion, chopped

1 large tomato, chopped

1 carrot, finely chopped

1 large handful of fresh basil, chopped

600mls (1 pint) vegetable stock (broth)

600mls (1 pint) hot water

1 tablespoon olive oil

Sea salt

Freshly ground black pepper

SERVES 4

98 calories per serving

Method

Heat the oil in a saucepan. Add the onion, carrot and garlic and cook for 3 minutes. Add in the tomato and red peppers (bell peppers), hot water and stock and cook for 10 minutes. Add in the basil. Using a hand blender or food processor, blitz the soup until smooth. Season with salt and pepper. Serve and enjoy.

Fast Tomato Soup

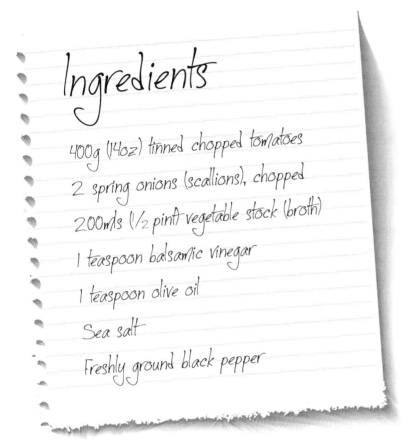

Ingredients

400g (14oz) tinned chopped tomatoes

2 spring onions (scallions), chopped

200mls (½ pint) vegetable stock (broth)

1 teaspoon balsamic vinegar

1 teaspoon olive oil

Sea salt

Freshly ground black pepper

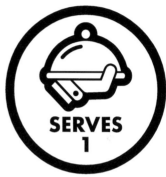

SERVES 1

133
calories
per serving

Method

Heat the oil in a saucepan, add the spring onions (scallion) and cook for 2 minutes. Add in the tomatoes and stock (broth) and bring it to the boil. Add in a teaspoon of balsamic vinegar. Reduce the heat and simmer for 5 minutes until heated through. Using a food processor and or hand blender blitz until smooth. Season with salt and pepper. Enjoy.

Serrano & Rocket Salad

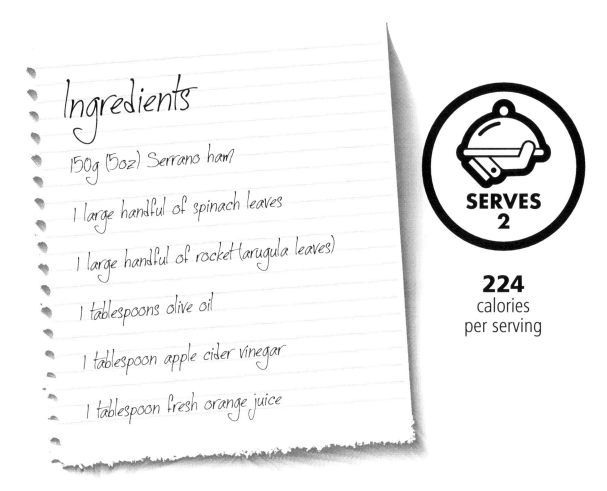

Ingredients

150g (5oz) Serrano ham

1 large handful of spinach leaves

1 large handful of rocket (arugula leaves)

1 tablespoons olive oil

1 tablespoon apple cider vinegar

1 tablespoon fresh orange juice

SERVES 2

224 calories per serving

Method

Pour the oil, vinegar and juice into a bowl and toss the spinach and rocket (arugula) leaves in the mixture. Serve the leaves onto plates and place the ham on top.

Lentil Soup

Ingredients

400g (14oz) tin of chopped tomatoes

350g (12oz) tinned green lentils (drained)

1 onion, chopped

1 teaspoon ground cumin

1 tablespoon olive oil

900mls (1½ pints) hot vegetable stock (broth)

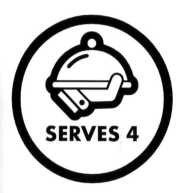

SERVES 4

168
calories
per serving

Method

Heat the oil in a frying pan, add the onion and cook for 4 minutes. Add in the vegetable stock (broth), tomatoes, lentils and cumin and bring it to a simmer for around 5 minutes. Use a hand blender or food processor and blitz until smooth. Serve and enjoy.

Gazpacho

Ingredients

10 tomatoes, de-seeded and chopped

5 cloves of garlic, chopped

2 red peppers (bell peppers), de-seeded and chopped

2 medium cucumbers, peeled and chopped

1 teaspoon chilli flakes

4 tablespoons apple cider vinegar

2 teaspoons olive oil

Sea salt

Freshly ground black pepper

SERVES 4

122 calories per serving

Method

Place all of the ingredients into a food processor or blender and blitz until smooth. If the soup is too thick, just add a little extra oil or vinegar. Eat straight away or chill in the fridge before serving.

Egg Drop Soup

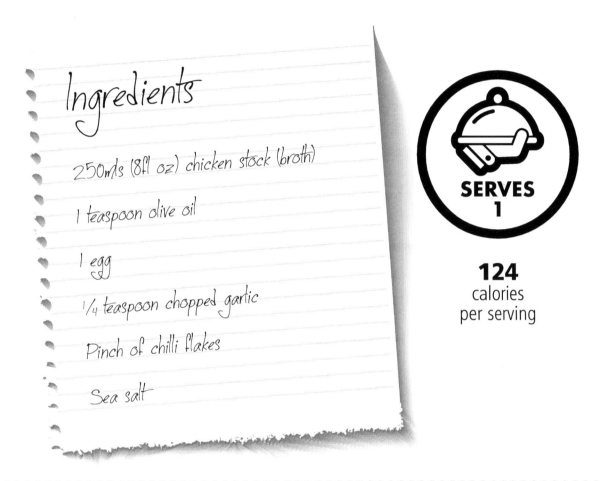

Ingredients

250mls (8fl oz) chicken stock (broth)

1 teaspoon olive oil

1 egg

1/4 teaspoon chopped garlic

Pinch of chilli flakes

Sea salt

SERVES 1

124 calories per serving

Method

Heat the oil and chicken stock (broth) in a saucepan and bring it to the boil. Add in the garlic, chilli and salt and stir. Remove it from the heat. In a bowl, whisk the egg then pour it into the saucepan. Stir for around 2 minutes until the egg is cooked. Serve and eat immediately.

Asparagus Soup

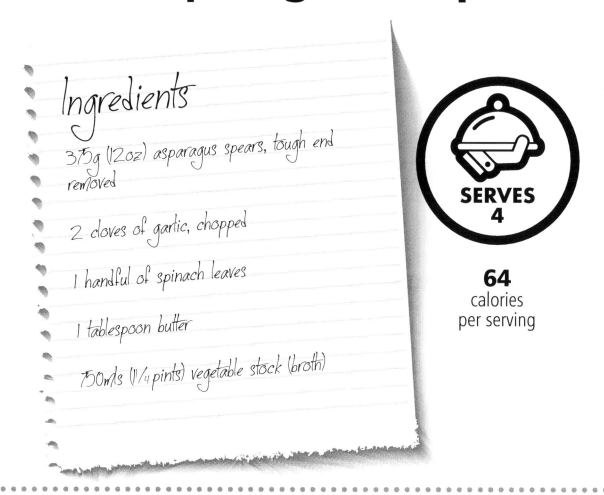

Ingredients

375g (12oz) asparagus spears, tough end removed

2 cloves of garlic, chopped

1 handful of spinach leaves

1 tablespoon butter

750mls (1¼ pints) vegetable stock (broth)

SERVES 4

64 calories per serving

Method

Heat the butter in a saucepan, add the asparagus and garlic and cook for 4 minutes. Add in the spinach and vegetable stock (broth) and cook for 5 minutes. Using a hand blender or food processor blend the soup until smooth. Serve into bowls.

Creamy Chicken & Vegetable Soup

Ingredients

275g (10z) cooked chicken (leftover roast chicken is ideal)

3 tablespoons crème fraîche

2 carrots, chopped (or you can use leftovers if you have them)

1 onion, finely chopped

1 tablespoon olive oil

1/2 teaspoon dried mixed herbs

1 litre (1 1/2 pints) vegetable stock (broth)

SERVES 4

188 calories per serving

Method

Heat the oil in a saucepan, add the onion, carrots and mixed herbs and cook for 4 minutes. Add in the stock (broth) and chicken and bring it to the boil. Reduce the heat and simmer for 4 minutes. Stir in the crème fraîche. Using a hand blender or food processor blitz HALF of the soup until smooth, then return it to the saucepan, making sure it is warmed through before serving.

Mediterranean Tomato & Lentil Soup

Ingredients

- 400g (14oz) tin of chopped tomatoes
- 350g (12oz) tinned cooked lentils (drained)
- 1 large onion, peeled and chopped
- 1 teaspoon dried mixed herbs
- 1 tablespoon olive oil
- 900mls (1½ pints) hot vegetable stock (broth)
- A large handful of fresh basil leaves, chopped

SERVES 4

148 calories per serving

Method

Heat the oil in a frying pan, add the onion and cook for 4 minutes. Add in the vegetable stock (broth), tomatoes, lentils and mixed herbs and bring it to the boil. Simmer for around 5 minutes. Stir in the basil. Use a food processor or hand blender and process until smooth. Serve and enjoy.

Turkey Soup

Ingredients

300g (11oz) cooked turkey (leftovers are ideal), cut into strips

200g (6oz) tinned chickpeas (garbanzo beans), drained

1 onion, peeled and chopped

1 red pepper (bell pepper), de-seeded and chopped

2 teaspoons ground coriander (cilantro)

2 teaspoons olive oil

1 handful of fresh basil, chopped

1½ litres (2¼ pints) vegetable stock (broth)

SERVES 4

242
calories
per serving

Method

Heat the oil in a large saucepan, add the onion and cook for 2 minutes. Add in the red pepper (bell pepper), ground coriander (cilantro) and stock (broth). Bring it to the boil, reduce the heat and simmer for around 6 minutes. Stir in the turkey, chickpeas (garbanzo beans) and basil and warm it through. Serve into bowls and enjoy.

Red Pepper & Cannellini Soup

Ingredients

- 200g (6oz) tinned cannellini beans, drained
- 1 onion, peeled and chopped
- 3 red peppers (bell pepper), de-seeded and chopped
- 2 teaspoons ground coriander (cilantro)
- 1 small handful of fresh oregano, chopped
- 1 small handful of fresh parsley, chopped
- 1½ litres (2¼ pints) vegetable stock (broth)
- 1 tablespoon olive oil

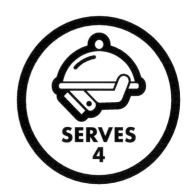

SERVES 4

140 calories per serving

Method

Heat the oil in a large saucepan, add the onion and cook for 2 minutes. Add in the red peppers (bell pepper), ground coriander (cilantro) and stock (broth). Bring it to the boil, reduce the heat and simmer until the vegetables have softened. Using a hand blender or food processor and blitz until smooth. Return it to the saucepan, add the cannellini beans, oregano and parsley and warm it. Serve and enjoy.

Celery & Blue Cheese Soup

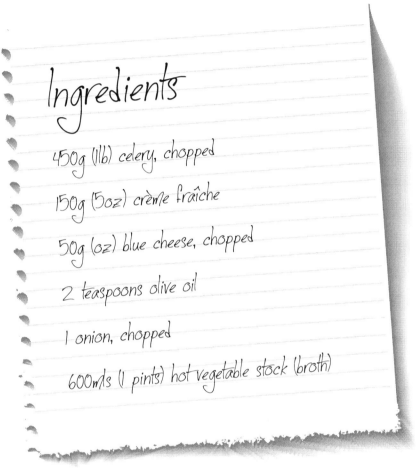

Ingredients

450g (1lb) celery, chopped

150g (5oz) crème fraîche

50g (oz) blue cheese, chopped

2 teaspoons olive oil

1 onion, chopped

600mls (1 pints) hot vegetable stock (broth)

SERVES 4

107 calories per serving

Method

Heat the oil in a saucepan, add the onion and celery and cook for 1 minute. Pour in the stock (broth), bring to the boil then reduce the heat and simmer for around 8 minutes. Add in the crème fraîche and stir in the cheese until it has melted. Serve and eat straight away.

Creamy Tomato & Pesto Soup

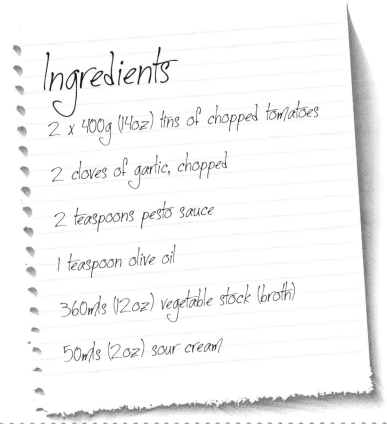

Ingredients

2 x 400g (14oz) tins of chopped tomatoes

2 cloves of garlic, chopped

2 teaspoons pesto sauce

1 teaspoon olive oil

360mls (12oz) vegetable stock (broth)

50mls (2oz) sour cream

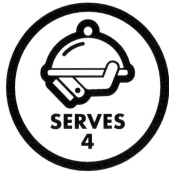

**SERVES
4**

70
calories
per serving

Method

Heat the oil in a large saucepan. Add the garlic and cook for 1 minute. Pour in the tinned tomatoes and vegetable stock (broth). Bring it to the boil then reduce the heat and simmer for 5 minutes. Using a hand blender or food processor whizz the soup until it becomes smooth. Serve the soup into bowls. Add in 2 teaspoons of pesto and a dollop of cream and swirl it with a spoon before serving.

Quick Chicken & Mushroom Soup

Ingredients

200g (7oz) cooked chicken, chopped

4 medium mushrooms, finely chopped

4 spring onions (scallions) finely chopped

2 stalks of celery, chopped

1 tablespoon olive oil

1 tablespoon crème fraîche

500mls (1 pint) hot chicken stock (broth)

Sea salt

Freshly ground black pepper

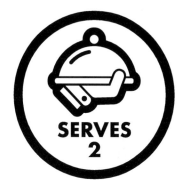

SERVES 2

239 calories per serving

Method

Heat the oil in a saucepan, add the mushrooms, celery and spring onions (scallions) and cook for 1 minute. Pour in the chicken stock (broth) and chopped chicken. Bring it to a simmer and cook for 8-10 minutes. Stir in the crème fraîche and season the soup with salt and black pepper. Serve and eat straight away.

Hummus With Carrot & Celery Crudités

Ingredients

- 1 carrot, cut into strips
- 6 celery stalks, cut into long strips
- 175g (6oz) tin of chickpeas (garbanzo beans), drained
- 2 cloves of garlic, crushed
- 1 tablespoon tahini (sesame seed paste)
- Juice of 1 lemon
- 1 tablespoon olive oil
- Sprinkling of paprika

SERVES 2

115 calories per serving

Method

Place the chickpeas (garbanzo beans), tahini (sesame seed paste), lemon juice and garlic into a blender and blitz until smooth Spoon the mixture into a serving bowl. Make a small well in the centre of the dip and pour in the olive oil and sprinkle on the paprika. Serve the carrot and celery sticks on a plate alongside the hummus.

Lemon & Pine Nut Asparagus

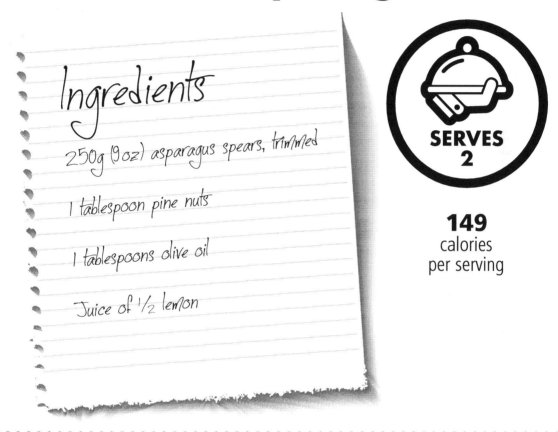

Ingredients

250g (9oz) asparagus spears, trimmed

1 tablespoon pine nuts

1 tablespoons olive oil

Juice of 1/2 lemon

SERVES 2

149 calories per serving

Method

Coat a griddle pan or frying pan with olive oil. Lay out the asparagus spears on it and squeeze the lemon juice on top. Cook for 6 minutes, turning occasionally. Scatter the pine nuts into the pan and warm them slightly. Serve and eat straight away.

Smokey Bean & Quinoa Salad

Ingredients

- 300g (11oz) tinned cannellini beans, rinsed and drained
- 300g (11oz) cooked quinoa, cold
- 2 large handfuls of fresh coriander (cilantro)
- 1 handful of fresh chives, finely chopped
- 1 teaspoon smoked paprika
- 1 tablespoon olive oil
- Juice of 1 lime
- Sea salt
- Freshly ground black pepper

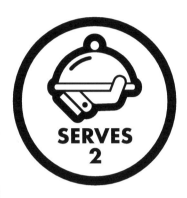

SERVES 2

378 calories per serving

Method

Place the beans, quinoa, coriander (cilantro), chives (scallions), paprika, olive oil and lime juice into a bowl and mix well. Season with salt and pepper. Chill before serving.

Beetroot & Lentil Salad

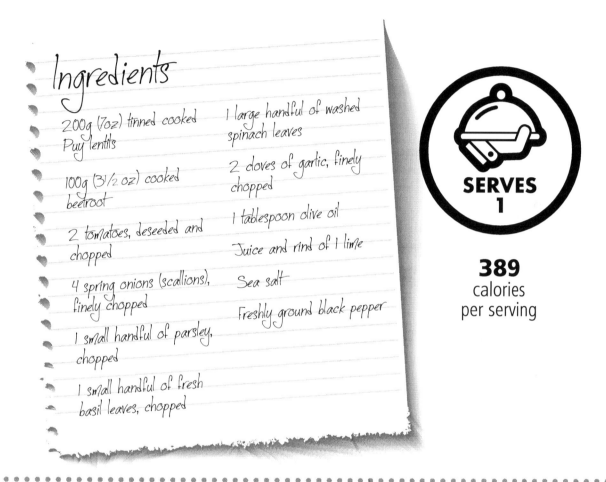

Ingredients

200g (7oz) tinned cooked Puy lentils

100g (3½ oz) cooked beetroot

2 tomatoes, deseeded and chopped

4 spring onions (scallions), finely chopped

1 small handful of parsley, chopped

1 small handful of fresh basil leaves, chopped

1 large handful of washed spinach leaves

2 cloves of garlic, finely chopped

1 tablespoon olive oil

Juice and rind of 1 lime

Sea salt

Freshly ground black pepper

SERVES 1

389 calories per serving

Method

Heat the olive oil in a saucepan, add the garlic and spring onions (scallions) and cook for 1 minute. Add the tomatoes, lentils, lime juice and rind. Cook for 2 minutes. Sprinkle in the herbs and stir. Scatter the spinach leaves onto plates, serve the lentils on top. Scatter the beetroot on top Season with salt and pepper.

Sweetcorn & Bean Salad

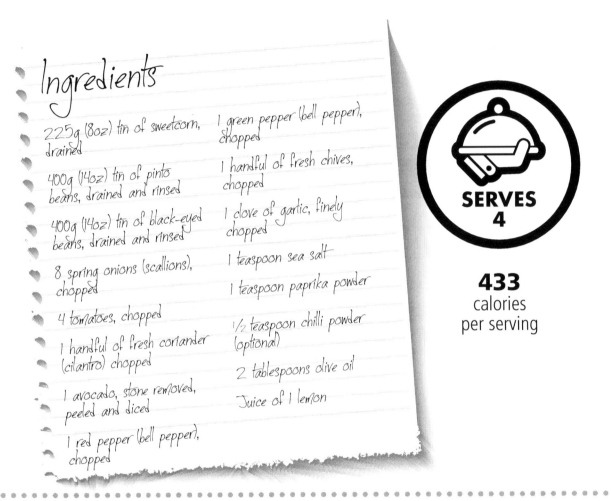

Ingredients

225g (8oz) tin of sweetcorn, drained

400g (14oz) tin of pinto beans, drained and rinsed

400g (14oz) tin of black-eyed beans, drained and rinsed

8 spring onions (scallions), chopped

4 tomatoes, chopped

1 handful of fresh coriander (cilantro) chopped

1 avocado, stone removed, peeled and diced

1 red pepper (bell pepper), chopped

1 green pepper (bell pepper), chopped

1 handful of fresh chives, chopped

1 clove of garlic, finely chopped

1 teaspoon sea salt

1 teaspoon paprika powder

½ teaspoon chilli powder (optional)

2 tablespoons olive oil

Juice of 1 lemon

SERVES 4

433 calories per serving

Method

Place the lemon juice, olive oil, paprika powder, garlic, salt and chilli in a bowl and mix well. In a large serving bowl, combine the beans, sweetcorn, avocado, tomatoes, peppers (bell peppers), spring onions (scallions), chives and coriander (cilantro). Pour the oil mixture over the salad ingredients and mix well before serving

Grapefruit & Pine Nut Salad

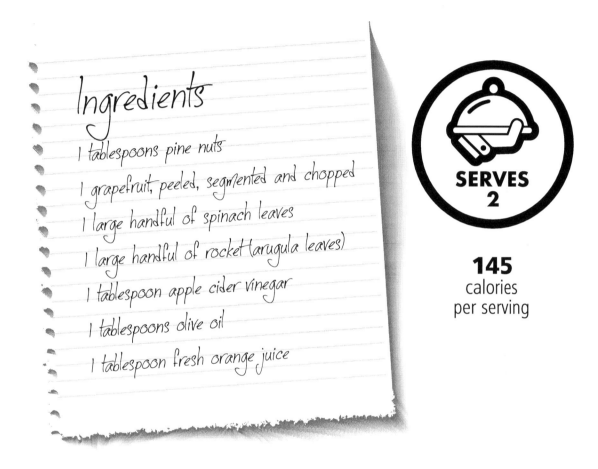

Ingredients

1 tablespoons pine nuts

1 grapefruit, peeled, segmented and chopped

1 large handful of spinach leaves

1 large handful of rocket (arugula leaves)

1 tablespoon apple cider vinegar

1 tablespoons olive oil

1 tablespoon fresh orange juice

SERVES 2

145 calories per serving

Method

Pour the oil, vinegar and juice into a bowl and toss the grapefruit, spinach and rocket (arugula) leaves in the mixture. Serve with a sprinkling of pine nuts. Enjoy.

Feta & Watermelon Salad

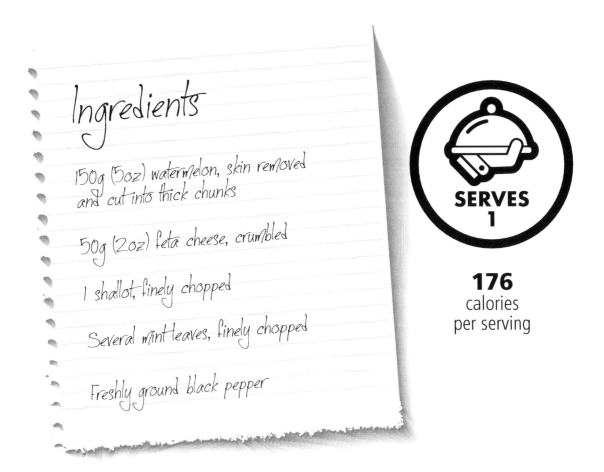

Ingredients

150g (5oz) watermelon, skin removed and cut into thick chunks

50g (2oz) feta cheese, crumbled

1 shallot, finely chopped

Several mint leaves, finely chopped

Freshly ground black pepper

SERVES 1

176 calories per serving

Method

Place the watermelon, shallot, feta and mint leaves in a bowl and mix to combine all of the ingredients together. Season with a little black pepper and serve.

Tuna & Cannellini Bean Salad

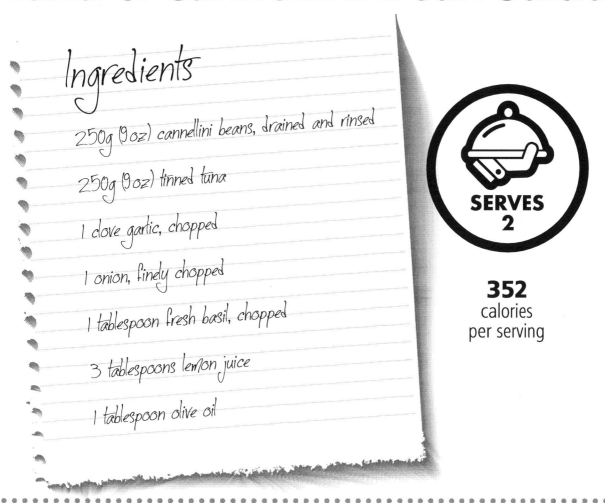

Ingredients

250g (9oz) cannellini beans, drained and rinsed

250g (9oz) tinned tuna

1 clove garlic, chopped

1 onion, finely chopped

1 tablespoon fresh basil, chopped

3 tablespoons lemon juice

1 tablespoon olive oil

SERVES 2

352 calories per serving

Method

Place the lemon juice, olive oil and garlic into a bowl and stir well. Add the cannellini beans, tuna, onion and basil to the bowl and coat them in the oil mixture. Serve and eat straight away.

Greek Chicken Salad

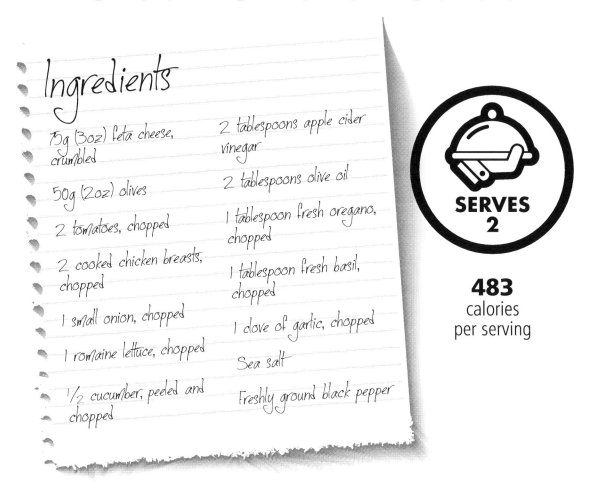

Ingredients

75g (3oz) feta cheese, crumbled

50g (2oz) olives

2 tomatoes, chopped

2 cooked chicken breasts, chopped

1 small onion, chopped

1 romaine lettuce, chopped

½ cucumber, peeled and chopped

2 tablespoons apple cider vinegar

2 tablespoons olive oil

1 tablespoon fresh oregano, chopped

1 tablespoon fresh basil, chopped

1 clove of garlic, chopped

Sea salt

Freshly ground black pepper

SERVES 2

483 calories per serving

Method

Place the oil, vinegar, oregano, basil, garlic, salt and pepper into a bowl and mix well. Add the chicken, lettuce, cucumber, tomatoes, olives, onions and feta cheese and coat the ingredients in the oil mixture.

Chilli Turkey & Avocado Salad

Ingredients

- 450g (1lb) turkey mince (ground turkey)
- 4 spring onions (scallions), chopped
- 2 Romaine lettuce, roughly chopped
- 2 tomatoes, chopped
- 1 red pepper (bell pepper), chopped
- 1/2 cucumber, chopped
- Flesh of 2 avocados, chopped
- 1 teaspoon chilli powder
- 2 teaspoons paprika
- 1 teaspoon mixed herbs
- 2 cloves of garlic, chopped
- 1 tablespoon olive oil
- Sea salt
- Freshly ground pepper

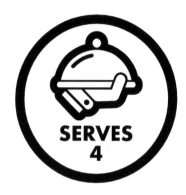

SERVES 4

344 calories per serving

Method

Heat the olive oil in a frying pan, add the turkey and cook until it's no longer pink. Sprinkle in the paprika, chilli powder, mixed herbs, garlic and stir for 2 minutes or until the turkey is completely cooked. Scatter the lettuce, avocado, cucumber, tomato, pepper (bell pepper) and spring onions (scallions) onto plates. Spoon some of the turkey mixture on top of each salad. Season with salt and pepper. Serve and eat straight away.

DINNER RECIPES

Surf & Turf Steak With Prawns And Garlic Sauce

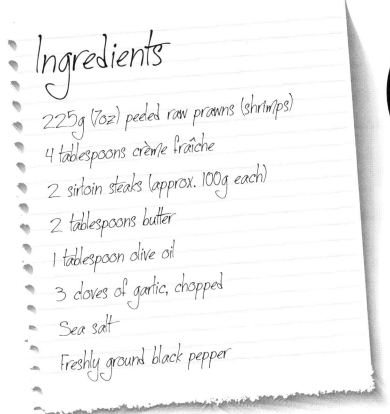

Ingredients

- 225g (7oz) peeled raw prawns (shrimps)
- 4 tablespoons crème fraîche
- 2 sirloin steaks (approx. 100g each)
- 2 tablespoons butter
- 1 tablespoon olive oil
- 3 cloves of garlic, chopped
- Sea salt
- Freshly ground black pepper

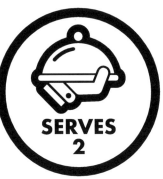

SERVES 2

400 calories per serving

Method

Sprinkle salt on each side of the steaks. Heat the oil in a frying pan, add the steaks and cook for 3-4 minutes, (or longer if you like them well done) turning once. Remove them from the pan and set them aside and keep them warm. Heat the butter to the pan, add the prawns (shrimps) and crème fraîche and cook for until the prawns are completely pink. Season with salt and pepper. Serve the steaks onto plates and spoon the prawns and sauce over the top. Eat straight away.

Chicken With Vegetable 'Spaghetti'

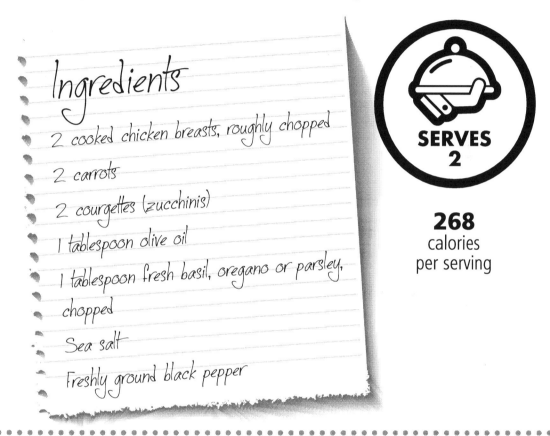

Ingredients

- 2 cooked chicken breasts, roughly chopped
- 2 carrots
- 2 courgettes (zucchinis)
- 1 tablespoon olive oil
- 1 tablespoon fresh basil, oregano or parsley, chopped
- Sea salt
- Freshly ground black pepper

SERVES 2

268 calories per serving

Method

Using a spiraliser, cut the carrots and courgettes (zucchinis) into strips. If you don't have a spiraliser, just use a vegetable peeler and cut into long then strips. Heat the oil in a frying pan, add the vegetables and cook for around 4 minutes. Add in the cooked chopped chicken and stir until it is warmed through. Season with salt and pepper. Sprinkle with fresh herbs and serve.

Tuna Steaks With Olives, Lemon & Basil Dressing

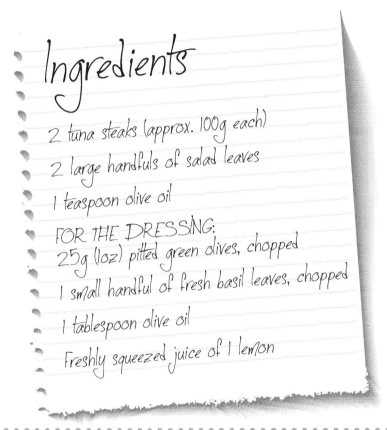

Ingredients

2 tuna steaks (approx. 100g each)

2 large handfuls of salad leaves

1 teaspoon olive oil

FOR THE DRESSING:
25g (1oz) pitted green olives, chopped

1 small handful of fresh basil leaves, chopped

1 tablespoon olive oil

Freshly squeezed juice of 1 lemon

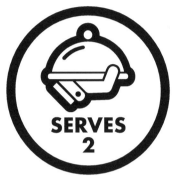

SERVES 2

235 calories per serving

Method

Heat a teaspoon of olive oil in a griddle pan. Add the tuna steaks and cook on a high heat for 2-3 minutes on each side. Reduce the cooking time if you want them rare. Place the ingredients for the dressing into a bowl and combine them well. Scatter the salad leaves onto plates. Serve the tuna steaks with the dressing over the top.

Quick Pesto Prawns

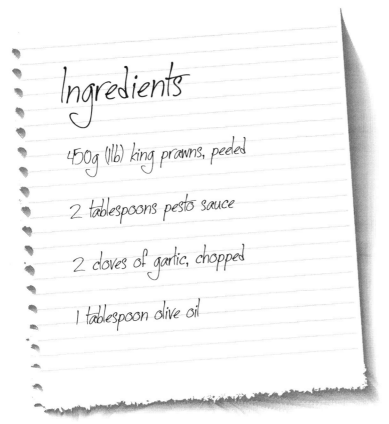

Ingredients

450g (1lb) king prawns, peeled

2 tablespoons pesto sauce

2 cloves of garlic, chopped

1 tablespoon olive oil

**SERVES
4**

154
calories
per serving

Method

Spoon the pesto sauce into a large bowl. Add the garlic and mix well. Coat the prawns in the pesto sauce making sure they are completely covered. Heat the oil in a frying pan, add in the prawns and cook for about 5 minutes until they are completely pink through. Serve on their own or with a green salad on the side.

Scallops & Pancetta

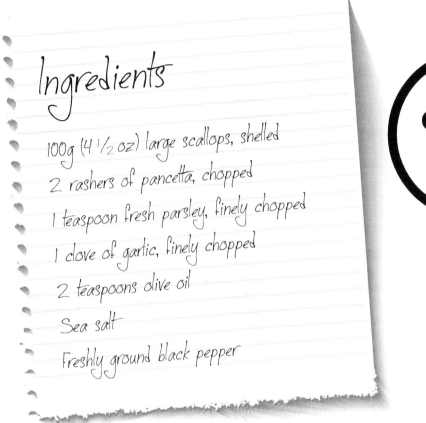

Ingredients

100g (4 ½ oz) large scallops, shelled

2 rashers of pancetta, chopped

1 teaspoon fresh parsley, finely chopped

1 clove of garlic, finely chopped

2 teaspoons olive oil

Sea salt

Freshly ground black pepper

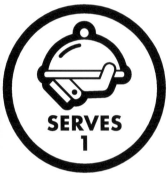

SERVES 1

240
calories
per serving

Method

Heat 1 teaspoon oil in a frying pan over a high heat. Add the scallops and cook for around 1 minute on either side until they are slightly golden. Transfer to a dish and keep warm. Add the pancetta to the pan and cook for around 2 minutes. Add a teaspoon of olive oil and garlic and cook for around 1 minute. Sprinkle in the parsley. Serve the scallops onto a plate and spoon the pancetta and garlic butter on top. Season with salt and pepper.

Pork Béarnaise

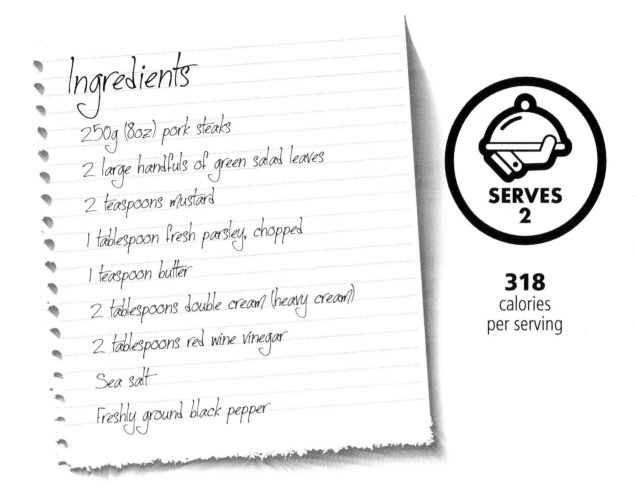

Ingredients

250g (8oz) pork steaks

2 large handfuls of green salad leaves

2 teaspoons mustard

1 tablespoon fresh parsley, chopped

1 teaspoon butter

2 tablespoons double cream (heavy cream)

2 tablespoons red wine vinegar

Sea salt

Freshly ground black pepper

SERVES 2

318 calories per serving

Method

Season the pork with salt and pepper. Heat the butter in a frying pan and add the pork. Cook for around 3 minutes on either side. Remove the pork, set aside and keep it warm. Reduce the heat and add in the vinegar, mustard and cream and stir well. Sprinkle in the parsley. Serve the pork onto a plate and pour the sauce over the top. Serve with green salad leaves.

Lemon Mustard Salmon & Lentils

Ingredients

- 250g (9oz) cooked Puy lentils
- 6 spring onions (scallions), chopped
- 2 salmon fillets
- 2 large tomatoes, chopped
- 1 small handful of basil leaves, chopped
- 2 large handfuls of rocket (arugula) leaves
- 2 teaspoons wholegrain mustard
- 1 teaspoon olive oil
- Zest and juice of 1 lemon

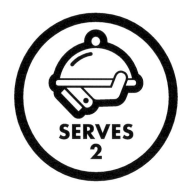

SERVES 2

399 calories per serving

Method

Place the lemon juice and mustard in a bowl and stir. Coat the salmon steaks in the mustard mixture. Place them under a hot grill (broiler) and cook for around 6 minutes turning once in between until the fish is cooked completely. Heat a frying pan, add in the oil, lentils, spring onions (scallions) and tomatoes and cook for around 3 minutes or until warmed through. Stir in the basil leaves at the end of cooking. Serve the rocket (arugula) leaves onto plates and serve the lentils on top. Lay the cooked salmon on top of the lentils.

Swordfish Steaks

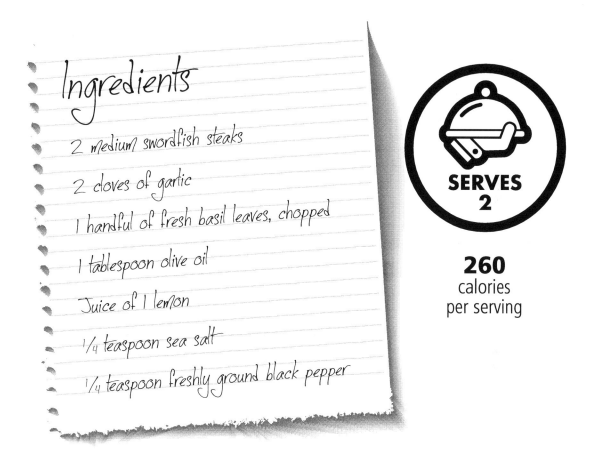

Ingredients

- 2 medium swordfish steaks
- 2 cloves of garlic
- 1 handful of fresh basil leaves, chopped
- 1 tablespoon olive oil
- Juice of 1 lemon
- 1/4 teaspoon sea salt
- 1/4 teaspoon freshly ground black pepper

SERVES 2

260 calories per serving

Method

Place the lemon juice, olive oil, garlic, basil, salt and pepper into a large bowl. Place the fish on a plate and lightly coat the swordfish with 1-2 tablespoons of the lemon oil mixture. Heat a little olive oil in a hot pan and add the swordfish steaks. Cook for 3-4 minutes on each side and check that it's completely cooked. Serve onto plates with the remaining dressing.

Pomegranate, Avocado & Chicken Salad

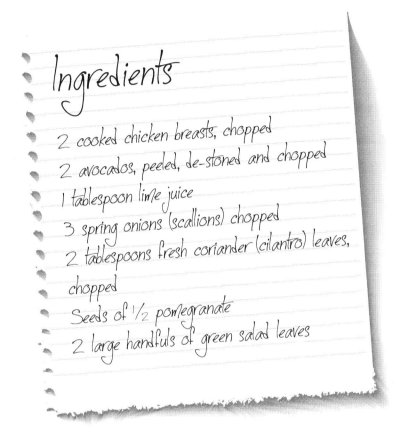

Ingredients

2 cooked chicken breasts, chopped

2 avocados, peeled, de-stoned and chopped

1 tablespoon lime juice

3 spring onions (scallions) chopped

2 tablespoons fresh coriander (cilantro) leaves, chopped

Seeds of ½ pomegranate

2 large handfuls of green salad leaves

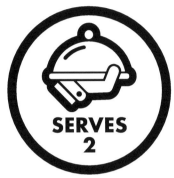

SERVES 2

423
calories
per serving

Method

Place the avocado flesh and lime juice into a bowl and mix well. Add the spring onions (scallions), chicken and coriander (cilantro) and mix well. Scatter the salad leaves onto a plate and spoon the chicken and avocado mixture on top. Sprinkle with pomegranate seeds. Enjoy.

Hazelnut Crusted Salmon

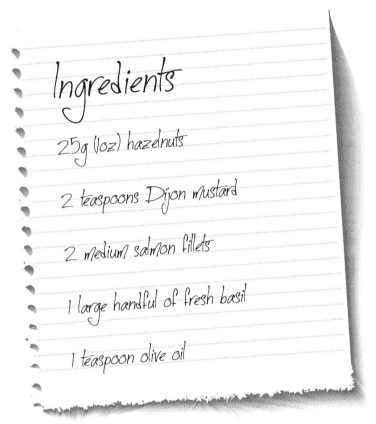

Ingredients

25g (1oz) hazelnuts

2 teaspoons Dijon mustard

2 medium salmon fillets

1 large handful of fresh basil

1 teaspoon olive oil

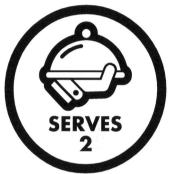

SERVES 2

387
calories
per serving

Method

Place the nuts, mustard and basil into a food processor and mix until soft. Heat the olive oil in a frying pan, add the salmon fillets and cook for 4 minutes on one side. Turn the salmon over and spoon the mustard mixture on top of the salmon fillets. Cook for around 3 minutes, or until the fish feels firm. In the meantime heat the grill (broiler). Finish the salmon off by placing it under the grill to finish off for around 2 minutes. Can be served alongside roast vegetables or a green salad.

Lamb Chops & Aubergine

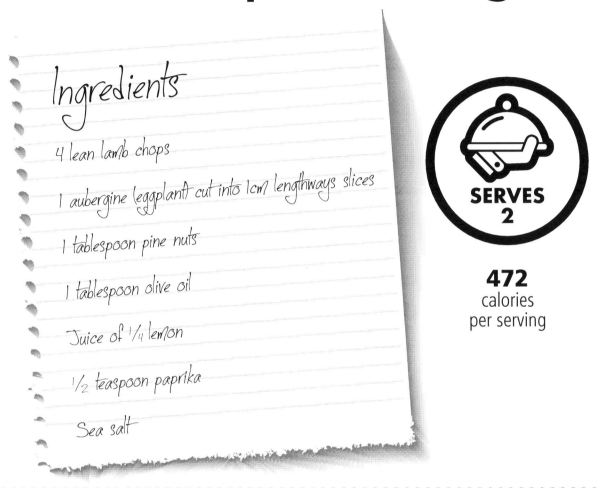

Ingredients

4 lean lamb chops

1 aubergine (eggplant) cut into 1cm lengthways slices

1 tablespoon pine nuts

1 tablespoon olive oil

Juice of 1/4 lemon

1/2 teaspoon paprika

Sea salt

SERVES 2

472 calories per serving

Method

Heat a griddle pan or frying pan on a high heat. Lightly coat the aubergine (eggplant) slices with oil and sprinkle with sea salt. Place them on the pan and cook until they soften, turning once halfway through. In the meantime place the lamb chops under a hot grill (broiler) and cook for around 4 minutes on each side or longer if you like lamb well done. Place the oil, lemon juice and paprika into a bowl and mix well. Serve the aubergine (eggplant) onto plates along with the lamb chops. Drizzle the dressing over the top and scatter on the pine nuts. Serve by itself or alongside a leafy salad.

The Essential 800 Calorie Mediterranean Diet
15 Minute Meals

Creamy Parmesan Chicken

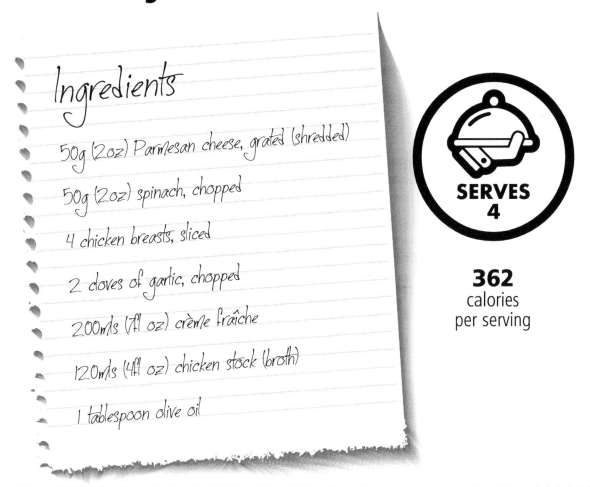

Ingredients

- 50g (2oz) Parmesan cheese, grated (shredded)
- 50g (2oz) spinach, chopped
- 4 chicken breasts, sliced
- 2 cloves of garlic, chopped
- 200mls (7fl oz) crème fraîche
- 120mls (4fl oz) chicken stock (broth)
- 1 tablespoon olive oil

SERVES 4

362 calories per serving

Method

Heat the oil in a frying pan, add the chicken and cook for around 5 minutes, stirring occasionally until it is cooked. Remove it and set aside, keeping it warm. Pour in the crème fraîche and add the garlic to the pan and stir. Add in the chicken stock (broth) and Parmesan cheese and stir until the mixture thickens. Scatter in the spinach and cook for around 2 minutes until it wilts. Return the chicken to the pan and make sure it is warmed through. Serve the chicken with the sauce. This goes really well with vegetable 'spaghetti'.

Sea Bass & Green Vegetables

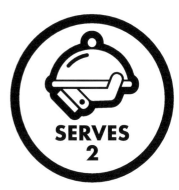

SERVES 2

249 calories per serving

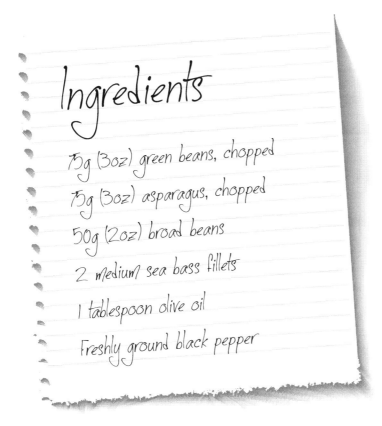

Ingredients

75g (3oz) green beans, chopped

75g (3oz) asparagus, chopped

50g (2oz) broad beans

2 medium sea bass fillets

1 tablespoon olive oil

Freshly ground black pepper

Method

Heat the oil in a frying pan. Add the sea bass and cook them for about 3 minutes. Turn them over and cook for around 3-4 minutes. In the meantime, place the green beans, broad beans and asparagus into a steamer and cook for 5 minutes until they've softened. Serve the vegetables onto plates and add the fish on top. Season with pepper. Enjoy.

Prawn, Avocado & Cannellini Salad

Ingredients

200g (7oz) cooked king prawns (shrimps)

150g (5oz) tinned cannellini beans

2 large handfuls of spinach leaves

1 avocado, peeled, de-stoned and chopped

1 teaspoon fresh coriander (cilantro) leaves, chopped

½ cucumber, chopped

½ teaspoon chilli powder

½ teaspoon paprika

Zest and juice of 1 lime

1 tablespoon olive oil

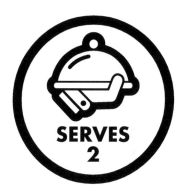

SERVES 2

373 calories per serving

Method

Place the prawns into a bowl and sprinkle on the paprika and mix well. Place the chilli, lime juice and zest and oil in a bowl and stir well. Add in the cannellini beans, avocado, cucumber and coriander (cilantro) and toss them in the dressing. Serve the spinach onto plates and add the tossed salad with the prawns on top.

Tomato & Herb Chicken

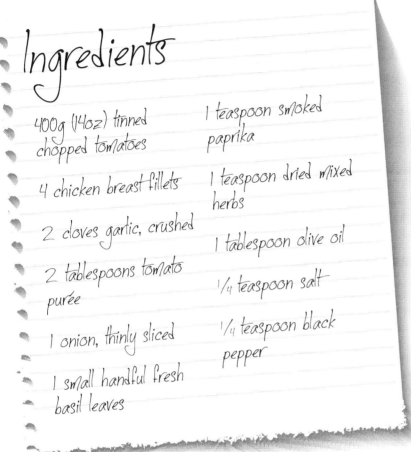

Ingredients

400g (14oz) tinned chopped tomatoes

4 chicken breast fillets

2 cloves garlic, crushed

2 tablespoons tomato purée

1 onion, thinly sliced

1 small handful fresh basil leaves

1 teaspoon smoked paprika

1 teaspoon dried mixed herbs

1 tablespoon olive oil

1/4 teaspoon salt

1/4 teaspoon black pepper

SERVES 4

227 calories per serving

Method

Place the chicken in a bowl and sprinkle on the paprika, salt and pepper, coating it well. Heat the oil in a frying pan, add the chicken and brown it. Add in the garlic and onion and cook for 2 minutes. Add in the tomato puree (paste), tomatoes and herbs. Bring it to the boil then simmer gently. Stir in the torn basil leaves and make sure the chicken is completely cooked before serving.

Creamy Turkey & Leeks

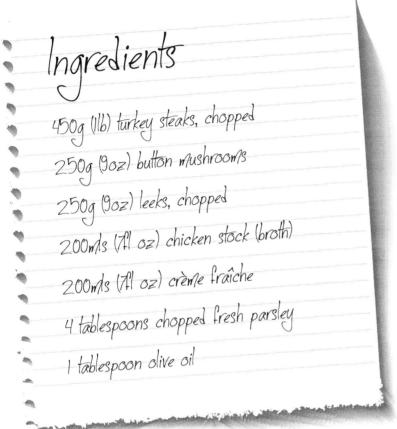

Ingredients

450g (1lb) turkey steaks, chopped

250g (9oz) button mushrooms

250g (9oz) leeks, chopped

200mls (7fl oz) chicken stock (broth)

200mls (7fl oz) crème fraîche

4 tablespoons chopped fresh parsley

1 tablespoon olive oil

SERVES 4

263
calories
per serving

Method

Heat the olive oil in a large pan and add the turkey and mushrooms. Cook for 2 minutes, stirring constantly. Add in the leeks and stock (broth) and cook until the vegetables have softened and the turkey completely cooked. Add in the crème fraîche and warm it through. Sprinkle in the parsley before serving. This is delicious with cauliflower mash.

Creamy Avocado 'Courgetti'

Ingredients

- 1 tablespoon pine nuts
- 1 medium courgette
- 1 ripe avocado, peeled and stone removed
- 2 cloves of garlic, peeled
- 2 teaspoons olive oil
- 1 teaspoon lemon juice
- 1/2 teaspoon paprika
- Sea salt
- Freshly ground black pepper

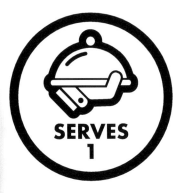

SERVES 1

466 calories per serving

Method

Use a spiraliser or if you don't have one, use a vegetable peeler and cut the courgette (zucchini) into thin strips. Heat 2 teaspoons of oil in a frying pan, add the courgette (zucchini) and cook for 4-5 minutes or until it has softened. In the meantime, place the avocado, garlic, paprika, lemon juice and a teaspoon of olive oil into a blender and blitz the mixture until smooth. Add the avocado mixture to the pan with the courgette (zucchini) and stir it well until warmed through. Season with salt and pepper. Serve and sprinkle with pine nuts.

Smokey Bean Casserole

Ingredients

400g (14oz) haricot beans, drained and rinsed

400g (14oz) pinto beans, drained and rinsed

400g (14oz) tinned tomatoes, chopped

200g (7oz) button mushrooms, halved

3 garlic cloves, chopped

1 onion, chopped

1 tablespoon smoked paprika

1 teaspoon chilli powder

1 large handful of fresh coriander (cilantro)

250mls (8fl oz) hot vegetable stock (broth)

1 tablespoon olive oil

SERVES 4

286 calories per serving

Method

Heat the oil in a saucepan, add the onions, mushrooms, garlic, chilli, beans, tomatoes and paprika and cook for 3 minutes. Pour in the stock (broth) and simmer for around 8 minutes or until the vegetables have softened. Stir in the fresh coriander and serve on its own or with rice, quinoa or potatoes.

Mustard Crusted Cod

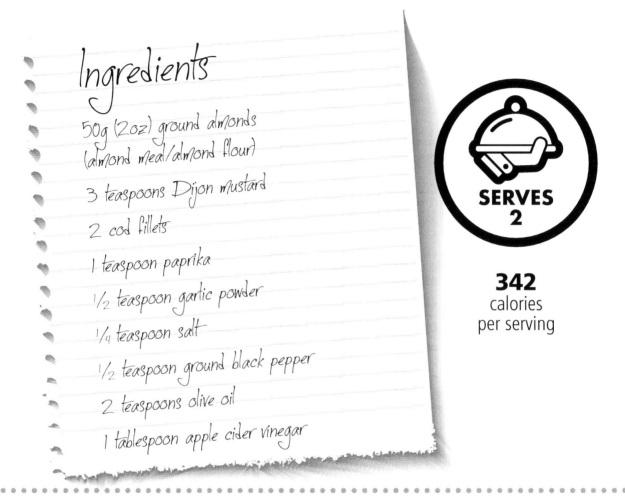

Ingredients

50g (2oz) ground almonds (almond meal/almond flour)

3 teaspoons Dijon mustard

2 cod fillets

1 teaspoon paprika

1/2 teaspoon garlic powder

1/4 teaspoon salt

1/2 teaspoon ground black pepper

2 teaspoons olive oil

1 tablespoon apple cider vinegar

SERVES 2

342 calories per serving

Method

Preheat the oven to 200C/400F. Place the almonds, paprika, garlic, salt and pepper into a bowl and mix well. Add in the mustard, olive oil and vinegar and mix well. Coat the cod fillets in the mixture. Place the fish on a baking dish and transfer it to the oven and cook for around 10-12 minutes or until the fish flakes easily. Serve the fish with green salad leaves. Enjoy.

Prawn & Chorizo Stir-Fry

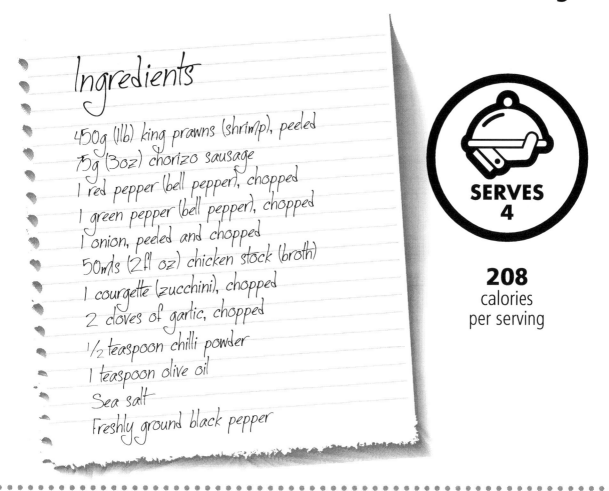

Ingredients

450g (1lb) king prawns (shrimp), peeled
75g (3oz) chorizo sausage
1 red pepper (bell pepper), chopped
1 green pepper (bell pepper), chopped
1 onion, peeled and chopped
50mls (2fl oz) chicken stock (broth)
1 courgette (zucchini), chopped
2 cloves of garlic, chopped
1/2 teaspoon chilli powder
1 teaspoon olive oil
Sea salt
Freshly ground black pepper

SERVES 4

208 calories per serving

Method

Heat the oil in a frying pan, add the prawns (shrimps) and cook for 3 minutes. Remove and set aside. Place the onion and peppers into a saucepan with the garlic and courgette (zucchini) and cook for 3 minutes. Add in the chorizo sausage and return the prawns to the pan. Cook for 2 minutes. Pour in the hot stock (broth) and add in the chilli. Season with salt and pepper. Make sure the ingredients are completely cooked. Serve and enjoy.

Asparagus & Red Pepper Sauce

Ingredients

25g (1oz) ground almonds (almond meal /almond flour)

14 stalks of asparagus, tough part of stalk removed

6 spring onions (scallions)

1 red pepper (bell pepper), halved and de-seeded

¼ teaspoon chilli powder

2 tablespoons water

1 tablespoon olive oil

Juice of ½ lemon

SERVES 2

177
calories
per serving

Method

Heat the oil in a griddle pan or frying pan. Add the asparagus and spring onions (scallions). Cook until they have softened, turning occasionally. In the meantime, place the red pepper (bell pepper), chilli powder, almonds, water and lemon juice into a blender and blitz until smooth. Serve the asparagus and spring onions onto plates and serve the sauce on the side.

Chicken & Green Peppers

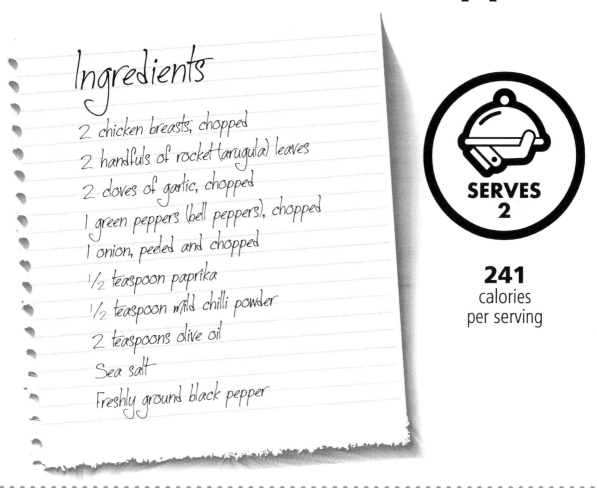

Ingredients

2 chicken breasts, chopped
2 handfuls of rocket (arugula) leaves
2 cloves of garlic, chopped
1 green peppers (bell peppers), chopped
1 onion, peeled and chopped
½ teaspoon paprika
½ teaspoon mild chilli powder
2 teaspoons olive oil
Sea salt
Freshly ground black pepper

SERVES 2

241 calories per serving

Method

Place the chicken in a bowl and sprinkle on the paprika and chilli making sure you coat it completely. Heat the oil in a large frying pan. Add the chicken and cook for around 3 minutes. Add in the onion, garlic, peppers and cook until the vegetables have softened. Scatter the rocket (arugula) on a plate and serve the chicken and vegetables on top. Season with salt and pepper. Eat straight away.

Garlic Prawns & Calamari

Ingredients

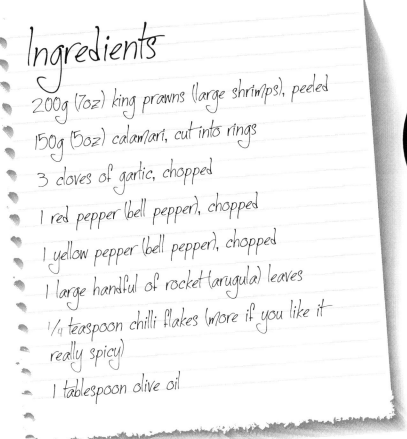

- 200g (7oz) king prawns (large shrimps), peeled
- 150g (5oz) calamari, cut into rings
- 3 cloves of garlic, chopped
- 1 red pepper (bell pepper), chopped
- 1 yellow pepper (bell pepper), chopped
- 1 large handful of rocket (arugula) leaves
- 1/4 teaspoon chilli flakes (more if you like it really spicy)
- 1 tablespoon olive oil

SERVES 2

244 calories per serving

Method

Heat a tablespoon of olive oil in a frying pan or wok. Add the peppers and cook for 3-4 minutes or until they have softened. Remove them from the pan and keep them warm. Add the garlic, prawns, calamari and chilli to the pan and cook for around 2-3 minutes or until the prawns are pink throughout. Toss the peppers into the pan and coat them in the juices. Serve onto plates and place some rocket (arugula) leaves on the side. Enjoy straight away.

Lemon & Basil Chicken Skewers

Ingredients

150g (4oz) chicken breast, cut into chunks

1 small bunch of basil, chopped

1 clove of garlic, chopped

Juice of ½ lemon

1 tablespoon olive oil

Sea salt

Freshly ground black pepper

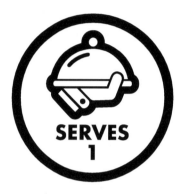

SERVES 1

357 calories per serving

Method

Place the oil, chopped basil, garlic and lemon juice in a bowl and mix well. Add the chicken to the marinade and stir well, covering the chicken completely in the mixture. Season with salt and pepper. Slide the chicken chunks onto metal skewers. Place them under a hot grill (broiler) or barbeque and cook for 5-6 minutes on each side or until the chicken is completely cooked through. Serve on its own or with salad and dips.

Aubergine Slices
& Houmous

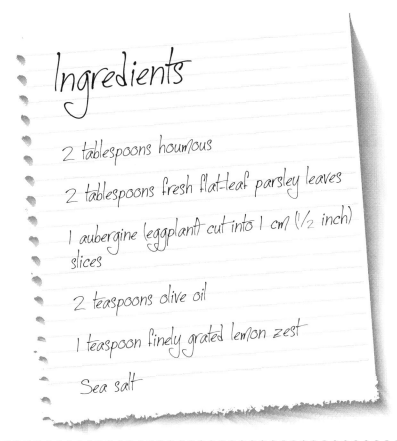

Ingredients

2 tablespoons houmous

2 tablespoons fresh flat-leaf parsley leaves

1 aubergine (eggplant) cut into 1 cm (½ inch) slices

2 teaspoons olive oil

1 teaspoon finely grated lemon zest

Sea salt

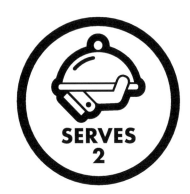

SERVES 2

249
calories
per serving

Method

Heat the oil in a large frying pan. Place the aubergine (eggplant) slices in the pan and season with salt. Cook for 3-4 minutes then turn the slices onto the other side. Place a small dollop of houmous onto each slice and cook for another 3-4 minutes. Serve onto plates with a sprinkling of parsley and lemon zest. Enjoy straight away.

The Essential 800 Calorie Mediterranean Diet
15 Minute Meals

Tomato & Mozzarella Skewers

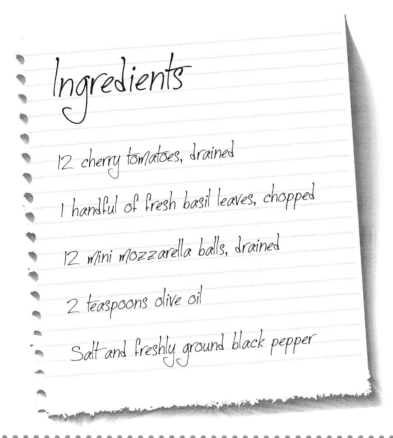

Ingredients

12 cherry tomatoes, drained

1 handful of fresh basil leaves, chopped

12 mini mozzarella balls, drained

2 teaspoons olive oil

Salt and freshly ground black pepper

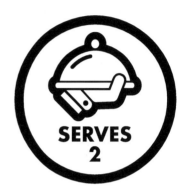

SERVES 2

318
calories
per serving

Method

Place the olive oil and chopped basil into a bowl and mix well. Add the mozzarella balls to the oil and coat them in the mixture. Thread the tomatoes and mozzarella alternately onto the skewers. Season with salt and pepper before serving.

Barbecued Mushrooms

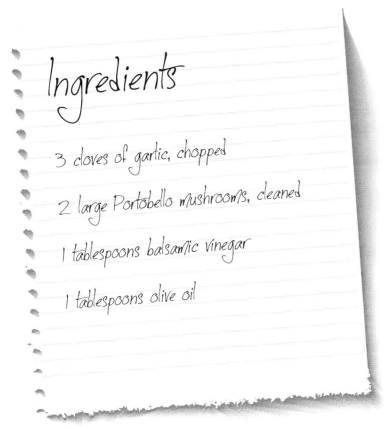

Ingredients

3 cloves of garlic, chopped

2 large Portobello mushrooms, cleaned

1 tablespoons balsamic vinegar

1 tablespoons olive oil

**SERVES
2**

90
calories
per serving

Method

Remove the mushrooms stalks, chop them and place them in a bowl. Lay the mushrooms with the gills facing up. Place the garlic, balsamic vinegar and olive oil in a bowl and mix well. Spoon the mixture into the mushroom cap. Cook them on a barbecue for 8-10 minutes.

DESSERTS, TREATS & SNACKS RECIPES

Passion Fruit & Raspberry Mascarpone

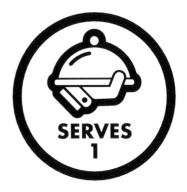

SERVES
1

235
calories
per serving

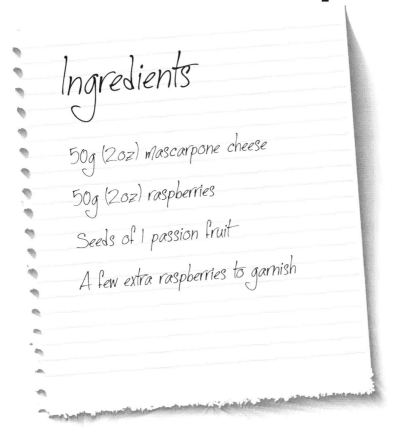

Ingredients

50g (2oz) mascarpone cheese

50g (2oz) raspberries

Seeds of 1 passion fruit

A few extra raspberries to garnish

Method

In a large bowl, stir the seeds from the passion fruit into the mascarpone and mix well. Place the raspberries in a separate bowl and mash them to a pulp. Using a tall glass or dessert bowl, spoon a layer of the mascarpone in then add a spoonful of the raspberry purée and swirl it slightly, repeat with another layer of mascarpone and raspberry until the mixture has been used up. Garnish with a few raspberries and chill before serving.

Iced Banana & Choc Chip Cream

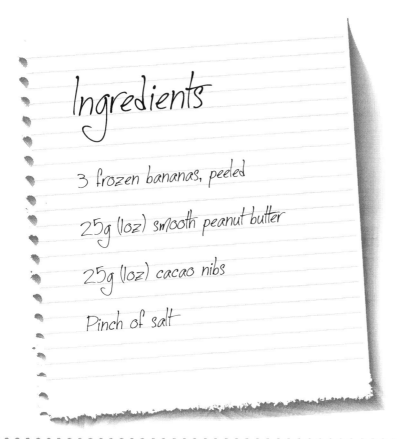

Ingredients

3 frozen bananas, peeled

25g (1oz) smooth peanut butter

25g (1oz) cacao nibs

Pinch of salt

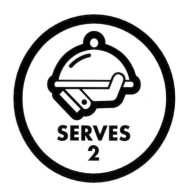

SERVES 2

276
calories
per serving

Method

This is a super quick dessert which does require you to freeze some bananas in advance.
Simply put the frozen bananas into a food processor and blitz until they become smooth.
Add in the peanuts butter, cacao nibs and salt. Blend all of the ingredients.

Apple & Caramel Dip

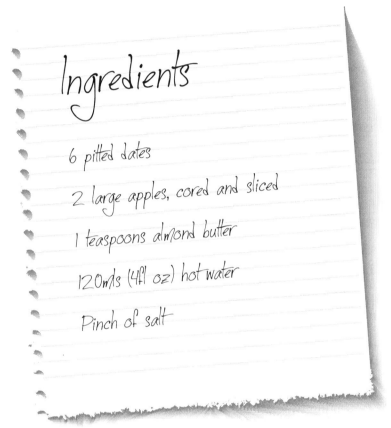

Ingredients

6 pitted dates

2 large apples, cored and sliced

1 teaspoons almond butter

120mls (4fl oz) hot water

Pinch of salt

SERVES 2

299
calories
per serving

Method

Place the dates, almond butter, water and salt into a food processor and combine them until the mixture is smooth and creamy. Spoon the mixture into a small serving bowl. Serve with the apple slices along with the dip.

Coconut Balls

Ingredients

125g (4oz) almond butter

75g (3oz) macadamia nuts, chopped

75g (3oz) desiccated (shredded) coconut

1 tablespoon tahini paste (sesame seed paste)

1 teaspoon vanilla extract

1 teaspoon stevia sweetener (or more to taste)

Extra coconut for coating

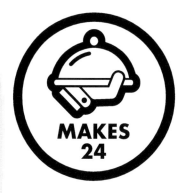

MAKES 24

80 calories each

Method

Place the coconut, tahini (sesame seed paste), almond butter, vanilla extract and chopped macadamia nuts into a bowl and combine them thoroughly. Stir in a teaspoon of stevia powder then taste to check the sweetness. Add a little more sweetener if you wish. Roll the mixture into balls. Scatter some desiccated (shredded) coconut on a plate and coat the balls in it. Keep them refrigerated until ready to use.

Cherry & Chocolate Milkshake

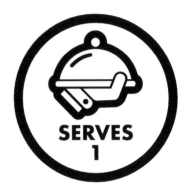

SERVES 1

233
calories
per serving

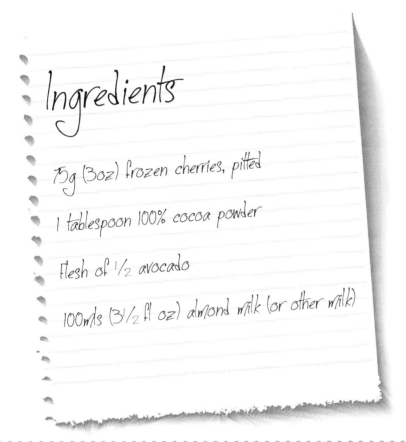

Ingredients

75g (3oz) frozen cherries, pitted

1 tablespoon 100% cocoa powder

Flesh of 1/2 avocado

100mls (3 1/2 fl oz) almond milk (or other milk)

Method

Place all of the ingredients into a food processor or smoothie maker and process until smooth and creamy. Serve and enjoy.

Banana Frappuccino

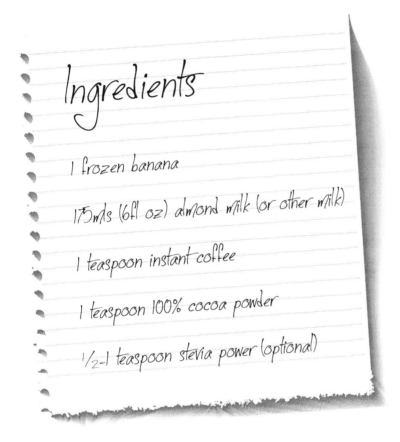

Ingredients

1 frozen banana

175mls (6fl oz) almond milk (or other milk)

1 teaspoon instant coffee

1 teaspoon 100% cocoa powder

½-1 teaspoon stevia power (optional)

**SERVES
1**

143
calories
per serving

Method

Toss all of the ingredients into a blender and blitz until smooth. Drink it straight away and enjoy!

Fruit Infused Water

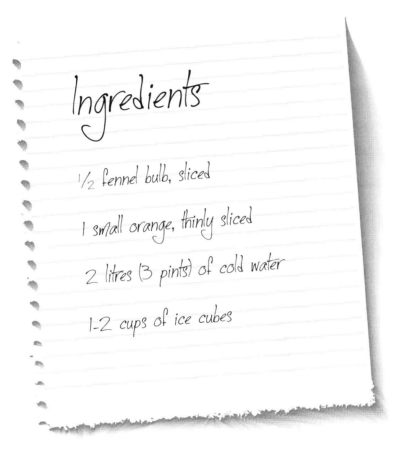

Ingredients

½ fennel bulb, sliced

1 small orange, thinly sliced

2 litres (3 pints) of cold water

1-2 cups of ice cubes

25
calories
per jug

Method

Fill a glass jug with water, add the fennel, orange and some ice and refrigerate it for 2-3 hours. You only also experiment with some of these tasty combinations.

Lemon & Ginger

Raspberry & Basil

Pineapple, Cherry & Lemon

Strawberry & Lime

Cucumber & Fresh Mint

Raspberry & Orange

Apple, Ginger & Cinnamon

Pineapple & Mango

Apricot & Raspberry

Cucumber & Lemon

Orange & Thyme

Mango & Lime

Kiwi & Lemon

Lime & Cucumber

Guacamole

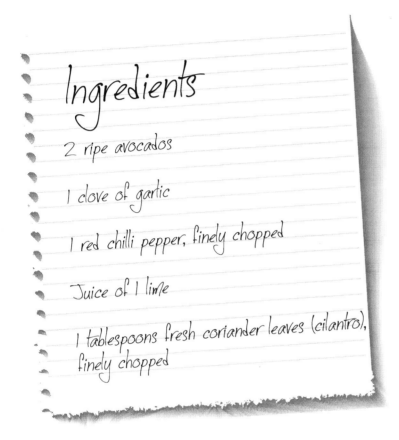

Ingredients

2 ripe avocados

1 clove of garlic

1 red chilli pepper, finely chopped

Juice of 1 lime

1 tablespoons fresh coriander leaves (cilantro), finely chopped

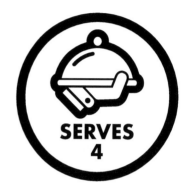

SERVES 4

140 calories per serving

Method

Remove the stone from the avocados and scoop out the flesh. Combine all the ingredients in a bowl and mash together until smooth. Garnish with fresh coriander.

Parmesan Kale Chips

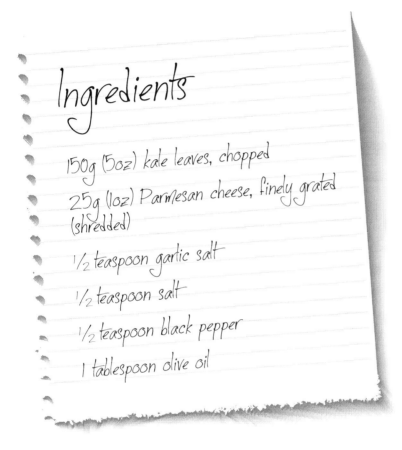

Ingredients

150g (5oz) kale leaves, chopped

25g (1oz) Parmesan cheese, finely grated (shredded)

1/2 teaspoon garlic salt

1/2 teaspoon salt

1/2 teaspoon black pepper

1 tablespoon olive oil

SERVES 4

66
calories
per serving

Method

Preheat the oven to 200C/400F. Line a baking sheet with foil. Scatter the kale leaves on the baking sheet. Drizzle the oil over the top and sprinkle on the Parmesan cheese, garlic salt, oil, salt and black pepper. Place it in the oven and cook for 8-10 minutes.

You may also be interested in other titles by
Erin Rose Publishing
which are available in both paperback and ebook.

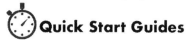 Quick Start Guides

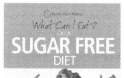
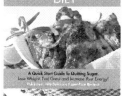

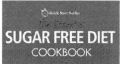
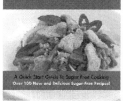

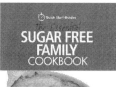
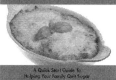

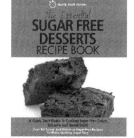

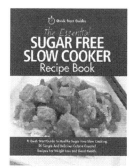
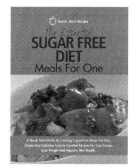
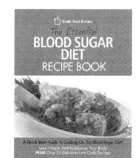
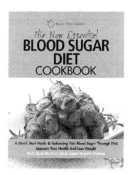

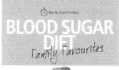
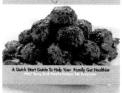
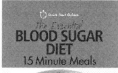
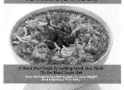
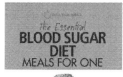
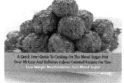
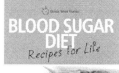
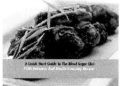

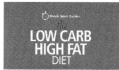
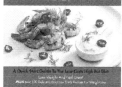
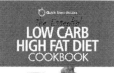
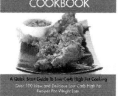
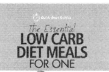
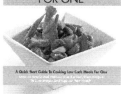
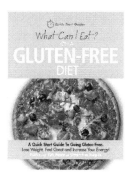

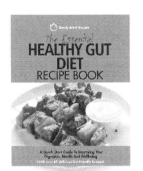
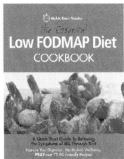
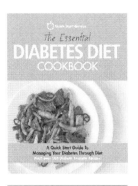
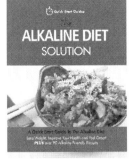
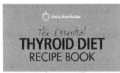
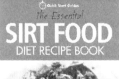
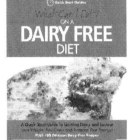
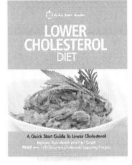
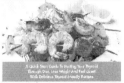
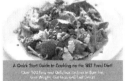
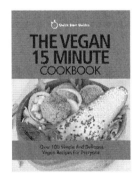
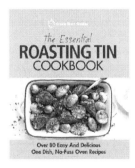
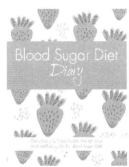
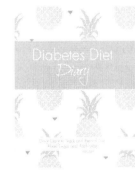
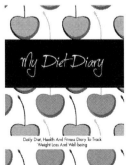
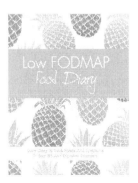
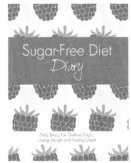
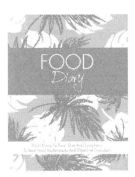

You may also be interested in titles by
Pomegranate Journals

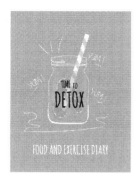
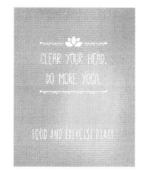
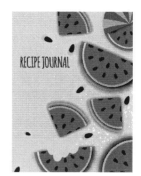
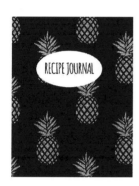
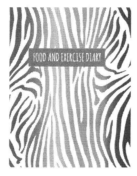
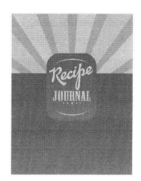
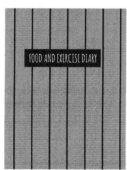
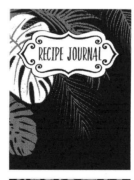
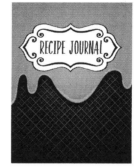
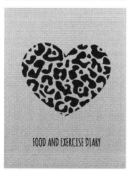
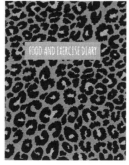
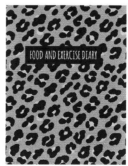

Printed in Great Britain
by Amazon